THE X FACTOR

WHAT IT IS & HOW TO FIND IT

The relationship between
inherited heart size and
racing performance

Marianna Haun

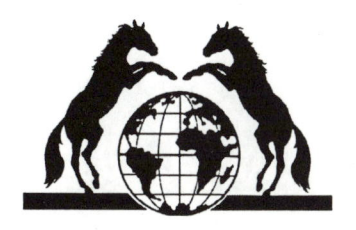

The Russell Meerdink Company, Ltd.
Neenah, WI 54956

Copyright 1997 © Marianna Haun. All rights reserved.

All rights reserved. No part of this book may be reproduced or transmitted in any form or by any means, electronic or mechanical, including photocopying, recording or by any information storage or retrieval system, without permission in writing from the publisher.

Library of Congress Cataloging-in-Publication Data

Haun, Marianna, 1945 -
    The X factor : what it is & how to find it : the relationship between inherited heart size and racing performance / Marianna Haun.
    Includes index.
    ISBN 0-929346-46-7
    1. Race horses--Genetics. 2. Heart--Size.
3. X chromosome. 4. Sex-linkage (Genetics)
5. Race horses--Speed.
    I. Title.
SF338.H38 1996
636.1'2--dc20   96-41931
                                                          CIP

Published by:

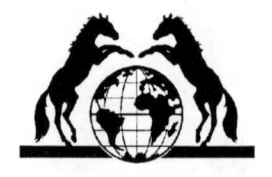

The Russell Meerdink Company, Ltd.
1555 South Park Avenue
Neenah, WI 54956
(414) 725-0955 Worldwide

Printed in the United States of America

To Secretariat,
whose great heart will race down
countless generations,
thanks to his daughters

Acknowledgements

Nothing worthwhile is ever accomplished without help. Among the people and farms who have helped with this project and book are: Dr. Frederick Fregin, whose knowledge and skill made all things possible; Dr. Gus Cothran, whose knowledge of genetics started the quest for the X Factor; Dr. Kathryn Graves for her expertise on the X chromosome; and Dr. Thomas Swerczek, who uncovered Secretariat's great heart.

Josephine Abercrombie, whose generosity in allowing us to measure her mares made the first steps of this journey possible; John Harris and Dave McGlothin of Harris Farms, whose generous support and unstinting help allowed us a large enough group of horses and family lines to really be able to follow the path of the large heart from sire to daughter to son and daughter; my daughter-in-law, Tina Baskins, a brilliant biologist, who took the time to help me understand genetics and my son, Kelly, who is always there for me; Penny Chenery for her gracious help; Henry White, whose help was always available; Associated Press sports writer, Mike Embry, the best editor a writer could have; Ed Bowen, who always listened; Keeneland Library's Phyllis Rogers and Cathy Schenck and the greatest equine research resources and racing negative collections in the world; Sharon Tolliver, whose Thanksgiving dinner in 1992 started the whole thing; Charlie and Bet Ketron, who were always there with support and sustenance; Patty and Terry Haun, whose visit on opening day at Keeneland inspired the book; and Jim Lane, who provided a Key to the Kingdom daughter.

The whole project wouldn't have been possible without the generous help of Kentucky farms such as Claiborne, Lane's End, Gainesway, Greentree, Ashford Stud, Calumet, Wood's Edge, Pin Oak, Plum Lane Farm, Crestwood Farm, Castleton Farm, Gold Springs Farm, Lanark Farm and Overbrook Farm.

CONTENTS

PART I
THE SEARCH BEGINS

Chapter 1   Great Heart   11

PART II
THE HISTORICAL AND BIOLOGICAL SEARCH

Chapter 2   The Start   17
Chapter 3   Human Athletes and Large Hearts   19
Chapter 4   The False Trails   23
Chapter 5   The Origin of Heart Score   27
Chapter 6   The Link Between Heart Score and
             Performance   33
Chapter 7   The 120 Heart Score Advantage   39
Chapter 8   Trotters and Heart Score   43

Part III
THE GENETIC SEARCH

Chapter 9   Searching for the Heart Score Genes   57
Chapter 10   The X Factor   65
Chapter 11   Champions and the X Factor   75
Chapter 12   Double Copy Mares   85

PART IV
THE GREAT LINES

Chapter 13	Princequillo	99
Chapter 14	War Admiral	111
Chapter 15	Blue Larkspur	117
Chapter 16	Mahmoud	121
Chapter 17	Large Hearts in Small Packages	125

PART V
PUTTING THE X FACTOR TO WORK

Chapter 18	Covering the Genetic Bases	133
Chapter 19	How to Measure Hearts	149
Chapter 20	Current Research	163
Chapter 21	Cher Chez la Femme	167
Epilogue	The Secretariat Story	169
Appendix	Heart Line Pedigrees	177
Index		198
Names in Pedigrees		202

FOREWORD

For the past two years the team of equine cardiologist, Dr. Frederick Fregin, Director of the Marion duPont Scott Equine Medical Center in Leesburg, Virginia; University of Kentucky geneticist Dr. Gus Cothran, University of Kentucky pathologist, Dr. Thomas Swerczek, University of Kentucky geneticist, Dr. Kathryn Graves, and writer Marianna Haun, discoverer of the X Factor, have been conducting heart measurements, collecting blood samples for DNA analysis and charting autopsies of Thoroughbreds from Kentucky to California. The purpose of the project is to document the sex linkage of the large heart characteristic and seek the genetic marker on the X chromosome.

The findings will be part of the equine genetic map currently under way at the University of Kentucky. University researchers are now looking for particular microsatellite variants or genetic markers that are always associated with the large heart. Because microsatellites are inherited from each parent, they can also be used as markers for genetic traits. So far, the researchers have found several sex-linked microsatellites on the X chromosome and are hopeful that they will help lead the way to finding the genetic marker for the large heart. If a microsatellite sequence is physically close to a gene of interest on a chromosome, that microsatellite can be used as a marker for that particular gene.

In this way, we can look at the inheritance pattern for a particular form of a gene, even though we don't know exactly what the gene is that is responsible for the phenotype in which we're interested. If DNA from individuals from at least three generations is available, the family can be screened by polymerase chain reaction (PCR) for the known microsatellites. If a specific allele of one of the microsatellites is found to be correlated with the large heart, that microsatellite is considered to be a marker for the gene controlling the trait.

In 1997, the team will conduct generational analysis studies using at least three generations of horses at Harris Farms in California, where there are families with at least three generations available for study. In depth pedigree analyses are also under way to prove the sex linkage of the large-heart characteristic.

PART I

THE SEARCH BEGINS

Chapter 1

Great Heart

In the spring of 1973, while the nation reeled from the revelations of Watergate, a hero emerged who captured the imagination of the country. He didn't come out of the halls of Congress, the White House, or Hollywood. He appeared on the racetracks of America - a big red colt - sweeping all before him, shattering records and galloping toward the first Triple Crown in 25 years.

On June 9, 1973, at Belmont Park, the "Big Red Machine," as turf writers had dubbed him, accomplished a feat that will be talked about for generations. As America held its breath watching the race on national television, the three-year-old Secretariat galloped away from the field to a 31-length victory to capture the third leg of the Triple Crown in the track record time of 2:24 for the mile-and-a-half Belmont Stakes.

Turf buffs can only wonder what his time might have been if there had been anyone to challenge him. Many who watched the race will long remember the announcer's amazed voice as he yelled, "My God, he's going to lap the field!"

Sixteen years later, that breath-taking race was explained. Suffering from a severe case of laminitis, Secretariat had been humanely destroyed. As the mighty stallion lay on an autopsy table at the University of Kentucky, a group of research pathologists surrounded him. As the veterinary pathologists began to cut into the stallion, they made a groundbreaking discovery: They uncovered the largest heart ever found in a Thoroughbred racehorse, estimated at 22 pounds.

The normal heart size of a Thoroughbred is 8.5 pounds.

The moment Secretariat was cut open and his great heart was revealed was a not only a record-making event akin to his 31-length record-breaking triumph in the Belmont Stakes, but it was truly a breakthrough event in heart research.

University of Kentucky pathologist Thomas Swerczek, in recalling the autopsy, said, "I had noticed a difference in heart size in horses during autopsies before we did Secretariat. I had picked up the difference in the male and females hearts and noticed that some were bigger than others.

"But I didn't pay much attention until Secretariat came along. He was completely out of everybody's league. Looking back to what he had done, it was easy to put a connection to it. The heart was what made him able to do what he did. It explained how he was able to do what he did in the Belmont - a mile and a half race. You would have to have a large heart to do what he did. It would be almost impossible for a horse with a small heart to do that."

After they had opened up the horse, the pathologists just stood there in stunned silence. Finally, one spoke up. "Now we understand that Belmont race," he said.

Dr. Swerczek, head pathologist at UK, who uttered those words, recalled the moment. "We just stood there," Swerczek said. "We couldn't believe it. The heart was perfect. There were no problems with it. It was just this huge engine."

Dr. Swerczek, the UK pathologist, said when they looked at the heart, they took it out along with the lungs.

"We took them out together and examined them," he said. "The lungs were not unusually enlarged. They appeared to be within the normal range. But when we examined the heart, clearly everything, the valves, the walls, everything was just perfect anatomically. There were no pathological lesions on valves or in the muscle.

"I looked at it microscopically. It was perfect. There was nothing wrong with it. It was just tremendously large."

Dr. Swerczek said that when the autopsy was performed there were more people present than was usual because of who the horse was.

"We did a routine autopsy, but we were careful. We didn't want to cut up too much of such a magnificent animal," he said. "I just couldn't make myself cut into his head, so we didn't examine the brain. People were there from the farm with plastic bags to make sure that every bit of the horse went back to the farm to be buried that day. That was the reason we didn't get an actual weight of the heart. In retrospect, that was one thing we should have done. I've seen thousands of hearts and this one was certainly unusual."

Among the other veterinarians at the autopsy was Clairborne veterinarian Walter Kaufman.

"After we exposed the heart, we all kind of looked at it and Dr. Kaufman turned to me and said, 'What do you think of the heart?' I said, 'It's humongous.' The other vets didn't have the benefit of looking at hearts every day, so they wanted my opinion. They obviously thought it was very large, also, but they wanted to make sure they were seeing what they thought they were.

"It is, by far, the largest heart I've ever seen. There is nothing to compare it with. The closest one was Sham's heart. I don't know how many years later it was that I did that autopsy (1993, 3 1/2 years later), but when I looked at it I immediately thought, 'My God, this is the second-largest heart I've ever seen.' But it was pathologically enlarged. It weighed about 18 pounds."

It was because of the weight of Sham's heart, which Swerczek could visibly see was smaller than Secretariat's, that he estimated Secretariat's heart weighed around 22 pounds.

Even in death Secretariat was still setting records. It was this discovery that would lead to further research on the large heart.

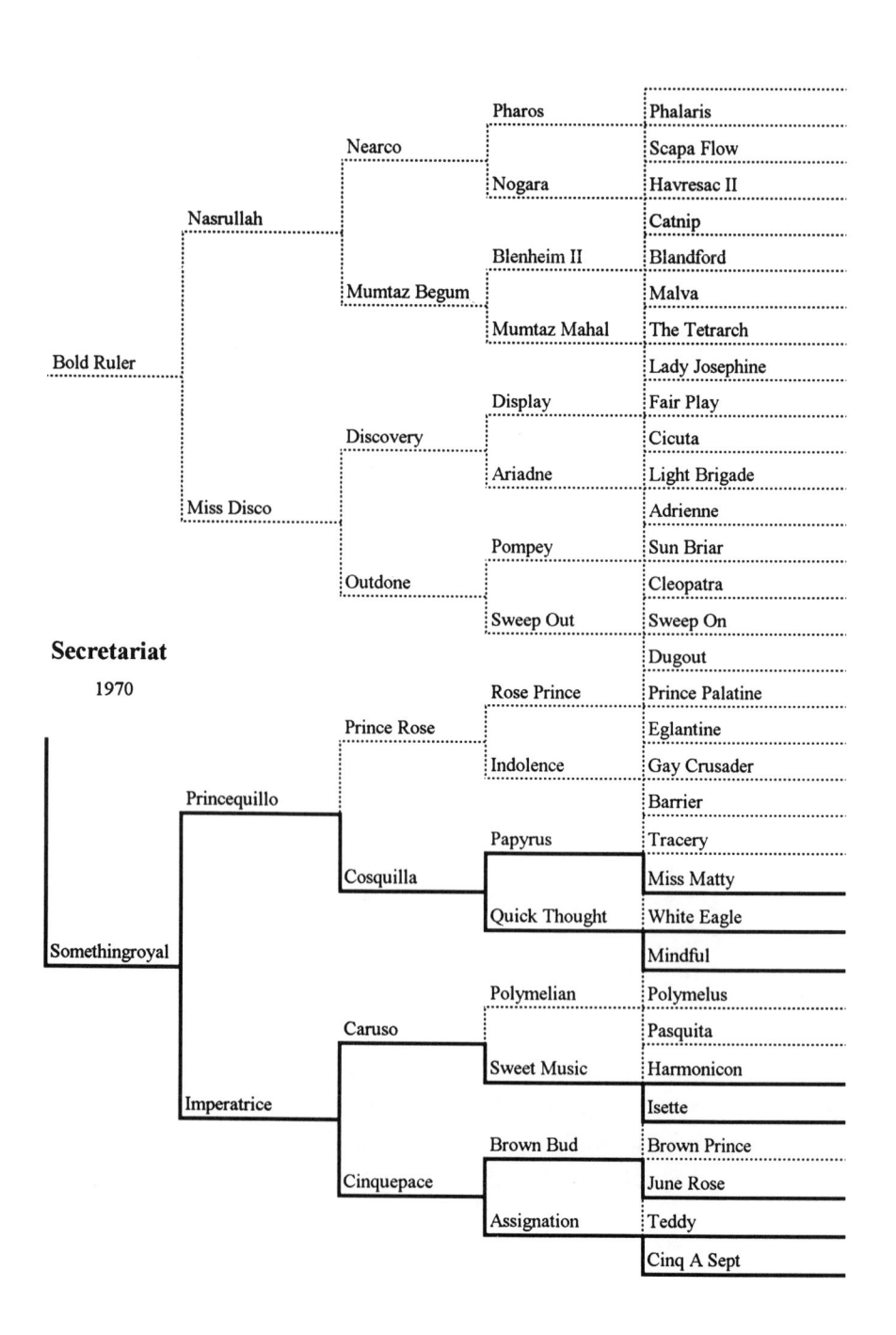

Secretariat
1970

Pedigree

Bold Ruler
- Nasrullah
  - Nearco
    - Pharos → Phalaris / Scapa Flow
    - Nogara → Havresac II / Catnip
  - Mumtaz Begum
    - Blenheim II → Blandford / Malva
    - Mumtaz Mahal → The Tetrarch / Lady Josephine
- Miss Disco
  - Discovery
    - Display → Fair Play / Cicuta
    - Ariadne → Light Brigade / Adrienne
  - Outdone
    - Pompey → Sun Briar / Cleopatra
    - Sweep Out → Sweep On / Dugout

Somethingroyal
- Princequillo
  - Prince Rose
    - Rose Prince → Prince Palatine / Eglantine
    - Indolence → Gay Crusader / Barrier
  - Cosquilla
    - Papyrus → Tracery / Miss Matty
    - Quick Thought → White Eagle / Mindful
- Imperatrice
  - Caruso
    - Polymelian → Polymelus / Pasquita
    - Sweet Music → Harmonicon / Isette
  - Cinquepace
    - Brown Bud → Brown Prince / June Rose
    - Assignation → Teddy / Cinq A Sept

PART II

THE HISTORICAL AND BIOLOGICAL SEARCH

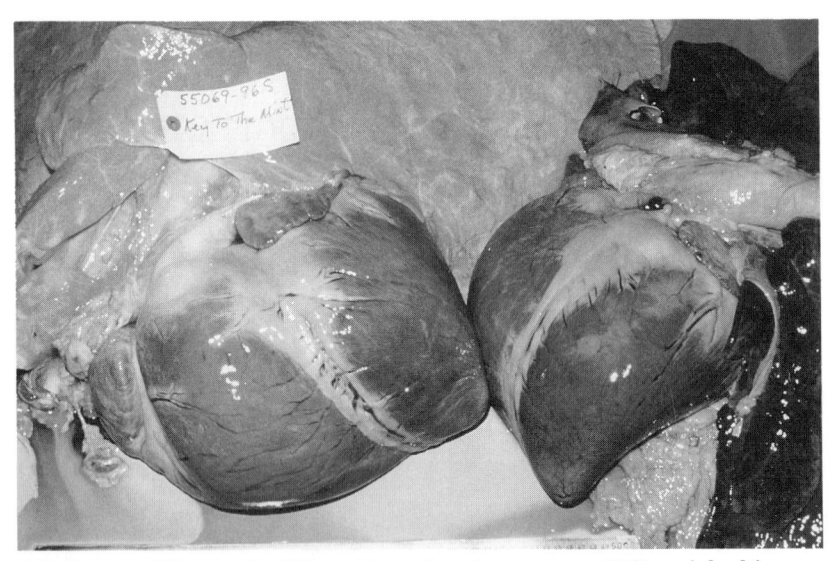

The heart of Key to the Mint, whose heart score was 157, weighed in at 15.8 pounds. It is shown here next to the 12 pound heart of another stallion.
Photo courtesy of Dr. Thomas Swerczek
University of Kentucky

Chapter 2

The Start

Until that 1989 autopsy, the racing world's benchmark had been the magnificent heart of Phar Lap, Australia's most famous race horse. So noteworthy was that great heart that it had been encased in glass since 1938 in the Australian National Museum in Canberra.

The 14-pound heart of the Australian champion gelding, foaled in 1926, has been preserved next to the 6-pound heart of an army remount horse. The size difference is staggering. Until the death of Secretariat, many felt that Phar Lap's heart was among the largest ever.

The pathologist who had performed Secretariat's autopsy, Dr. Thomas Swerczek, was called on, in 1993, to perform the autopsy on Secretariat's old rival, Sham. Three years earlier, while performing the autopsy on Secretariat, no one had thought to weigh his heart so there would be an exact size on record.

Because of this, Swerczek did weigh Sham's heart and it weighed 18 pounds. "I didn't weigh Secretariat's heart," Swerczek said, "but I could visually see that Sham's heart was smaller, so I estimated Secretariat's heart to weigh approximately 22 pounds."

It is one of history's ironies, that Sham, if he had foaled any other year would have been a champion, yet still had to finish second to Secretariat in death when it came to a great heart. He had finished second in the first two legs of the Triple

Crown, and in the third leg had challenged Secretariat to set that historic pace.

Penny Chenery, Secretariat's owner, remembers getting his autopsy and reading about her horse's huge heart. "I was surprised," she said, "that the heart was physically so unusually large. I had always believed in terms of emotion and courage it was certainly true. But its size explained to me how he was able to run a mile and a half in two seconds faster than anybody else. Watching him when he won the Belmont, you just couldn't believe what you were seeing. I remember being terribly relieved. He had done it. He had won the Triple Crown."

Chenery's reaction mirrored the traditional view of racing people. Surely, 'heart' was a characteristic of all the great champions. But was the term one which described a personality characteristic - something which was real but not measurable - or was it also a measurable physical attribute?

If it was real and measurable, could it be tracked and predicted? Or was it simply luck of the draw?

False trails and centuries of racing lore had served to cast a haze over the question. Surely, though, if a physically large heart could account for championship performance, it was a matter worth serious scientific investigation.

Chapter 3

Human Athletes and Large Hearts

There was already evidence from human biology.

Enlarged hearts have been found in human runners. Physiologist David L. Costill, who is a professor of exercise science at Ball State University in Muncie, Ind., and director of the university's Human Performance Laboratory, has written about the enlarged heart often found in outstanding distance runners.

Considered one of the world's top authorities in field of running, Costill wrote in his book, "Inside Running," that elite distance runners are known for their "efficient, and often enlarged hearts. The key to success in distance running rests on the capacity to deliver oxygen to the muscles. This task is the responsibility of the heart and arteries that serve as the oxygen transport system.

"The amount of blood that can be pumped out of the heart each minute (cardiac output) during exercise determines, in part, the capacity of the muscles to carry on aerobic energy production.

"Highly trained distance runners have frequently been described as having enlarged left ventricles, from which the heart chamber ejects the oxygen-laden blood into the arteries."

Costill reports on studies conducted in 1962 using the ECG to examine heart function and the size of hearts found in marathon runners at the British Commonwealth Games. In this study, it was noted that the runners had high voltage from the left ventricle (QRS complex) which indicated a large heart. In 1966, similar studies were conducted on 46 endurance athletes which demonstrated a high percentage of them had enlarged hearts.

Physical evidence of this was demonstrated with an X-ray of Paavo Nurmi, seven-time Olympic champion distance runner. The X-ray of Nurmi was compared with the X-ray of another man with a normal heart size. Nurmi's heart was nearly three times larger than the normal heart.

The contrast between another champion runner and an ordinary man was also confirmed when world champion marathon runner Hal Higdon's heart was compared with another man's heart of the same age, height, and weight. Higdon's heart was 50 percent larger than the untrained man's heart.

Costill also reports on the post-mortem examination of marathon runner Clarence DeMar, who won the Boston Marathon seven times and competed in more than 1,000 long-distance races. The autopsy revealed that DeMar had a significantly enlarged heart with relatively clean arteries.

DeMar was diagnosed with intestinal cancer, but he continued to train until two weeks before his death. When his heart was examined after death, it was found to weigh 340 grams, compared to the normal male heart weight of approximately 300 grams. The left ventricle wall was 18 millimeters thick, compared to a normal thickness of 10-to-12 millimeters, and the right wall was eight millimeters thick, compared to the normal thickness of 3-to-4 millimeters. Although the valves of his heart were normal, the coronary arteries were estimated to be three-to-four times larger than normal size.

Human biology, however, is not equine biology.

But there were other clues from other species. The greyhound racing industry had looked at heart size in dogs. A scientific paper published several years ago asserted a genetic connection in heart size in greyhounds.

It was, moreover, well established that the X chromosomes seem to have the same set of genes from marsupials to humans. This means that anything found on the

X chromosome in terms of heart can be translated into human heart research or any other species of mammals, including horses.

The importance of this finding for equine research was contingent on establishing that there was a real, quantifiable connection between heart size and performance. More importantly, it would only have a major impact on predicting equine performance if the genetic connection existed and could be traced in the bloodlines of the great horses.

Heart size and performance had to be correlated, surely. But more importantly, for predictive purposes, heart size had to be an inheritable trait.

Two factors stood in the way of the research.

First, it was clear that there had been great horses with normal size hearts.

But a greater obstacle was the long standing tradition in the racing community which placed almost all of the credit for great performance on the sire. The dam's influence was rarely considered to be of much importance.

Perhaps that bias is most easily explained by the obvious. And it is obvious that a sire can produce far more offspring than a dam. The data is more quickly available from a sire than a dam.

Chapter 4

The False Trails

That first obstacle was easily overcome.

That there had been great champions with normal size hearts was not open to question. Bold Ruler and Caro were perhaps the best known examples. Both had been found to have normal size hearts at autopsy.

In every area of endeavor, equine and human, however, there have been individuals who have had such superb characteristics in other areas as to make up for a lack in one area. Just as there can be an excellent basketball player who is not tall, there can be great horses with normal size hearts.

Further, the opposite side of the coin is just as true. The presence of a large heart in a racehorse has never been a guarantee of a winner. It is only a piece of the puzzle. There are too many variable in racing for one characteristic to be the "smoking gun" for a champion.

Heart size will not help a racehorse be a champion if he is unsound, has bad conformation, is not interested in running, is poorly trained, or any number of factors that can impact on the success or failure of a racehorse.

Dr. Anthony Stewart, a leading researcher in equine cardiology has conducted his own breeding studies using Thoroughbreds to breed for larger hearts. He personally uses heart scores when buying or breeding racehorses.

"I use the heart score as the final test when picking a horse," said Stewart, who is past president of the Victoria Racing Club. "Otherwise you end up with a lot of horses with big hearts that can't run. If you select on the basis of pedigree and performance and then you check the heart score and as long as the heart score is right you can say. . .'That will work.'

The greater obstacle to serious investigation was the emphasis placed by the entire racing community on the sire, rather than the dam.

Sexism has figured for centuries in the breeding of racehorses, with the arbitrary assignment of strong characteristics to the male side and the weak characteristics to the female side.

The dosage system, long in vogue, gives primary importance to the sire line, basing most of the hopes of breeders on the tiny Y chromosome.

Geneticist William E. Jones of California, wrote in his book, "*Genetics and Horse Breeding*," about the dosage system developed in the 1920s by Colonel Vuillier. The dosage system was described by Vuillier in the French publication, *Les Croisements Rationnels.*

As Jones described it in his book, "He had analyzed the pedigrees of many of the better Thoroughbreds of the time and found a relationship in the balance of blood of certain progenitors in them. Like prescription medicine, there was a dose of this and a dose of that. Colonel Vuillier computed that 15 stallions and one mare (Pocahontas) appeared in pedigrees of first-class horses with approximately the same frequency."

Because pedigree experts had more or less ignored the bottom side of the pedigree for years, Jones did not know why Vuillier included Pocahontas in his dosage system. These experts, Jones said, always clung to the idea that the sire line was the most important.

This belief is one of the reasons that Jones does not put much stock in the dosage system.

"When no credit at all is given to the mare, it is not many generations before a famous ancestor has no more than 'paper potency,'" Jones said. "At this point a breeder who believes strongly in dosage may argue that the mares all have sires, and that the influence of these sires is also figured into the system. This may sound like a good argument, but very few dosage proponents can show a system where the sire of the dams all the way back in the pedigree are calculated.

"The genetic makeup of a sire line is ever-changing. After 50 years of breeding, there will be no resemblance whatsoever to the original line. The sire line does not have the X chromosome going for it as does the tail-female line. The male chromosome (Y) carries so few genes that their significance is negligible," he said.

University of Kentucky geneticist Gus Cothran has also been bothered by the sexism in the dosage system and that displayed by many pedigree experts.

"I've always wondered how they could ignore half of the horse - the dam's side," Cothran said.

"It makes sense if you think of our culture. Science is frequently colored by the culture. That is what stays. The science involved in horse breeding has never been truly a science - it has also been the culture. So much of what we see accepted as scientific fact really comes from lay people who have not studied genetics.

"Way back when they started developing the Thoroughbred breed, they didn't know about genetics. They thought there was a blending. Certain characteristics coming from the male would be dominant because they thought the male was stronger. Because the male was stronger, his genes would be stronger. Because they didn't really understand the actual physical mechanism, they made a lot of incorrect assumptions. Because of tradition, many of these assumptions are still being used mistakenly today. Genetics is still a mystery to a lot of people currently involved in horse breeding."

"The principle of the X Factor has answered a lot of questions that I have had over the years about the dam's side of the pedigree," said Henry White, noted pedigree expert and advisor. "But the information is like a good hoe. It can get the job done, but it is no better than the user."

The stage, then, is set for a series of critical questions:

Is a large heart an important contributing factor in the performance of a great champion?

To answer that question, we need to know first whether a significant number of the great champions did, indeed, have large hearts.

That is the historical question.

If those large hearts were present, did they contribute significantly to the performance of those champions?

To properly answer that question we need to explore the mechanism of the heart - that 'engine' in Secretariat that had so amazed Dr. Swerczek. How does it work?

That is the biological question.

Only then can the most important questions be asked:

Where does that great heart come from?

Can it be predicted and planned for?

That was a question for genetics.

The trail begins with the historical question.

Chapter 5

The Origin of "Heart Score"

For centuries, the racing fraternity has looked for ways of determining how well a horse will perform. There are those who have placed all their credence in the horse's conformation, and those for whom breeding is the only factor worth considering. The list of attributes which have been thought to be critical have changed with fashion and with the visible attributes of the latest champion.

There has never been, perhaps never will be, a definitive answer to the question of what makes a champion. There are too many variables and too many ways to combine them. It is possible to say, though, that certain attributes seem to show up with regularity in the great champions.

One such attribute is clearly a large heart. Secretariat and Sham both had this physical attribute.

Historically, the fabled Eclipse, foaled more than 200 years before Secretariat, was found to have an extraordinarily large heart when he was cut open to have the traditional burial for great racehorses of just his heart, hooves, testicles and ears. The great Australian stallion, Star Kingdom, foaled in 1946, was found to have a 14 pound heart - equal to the reported size of Eclipse's heart. The great Mill Reef had been found to have a 17 pound heart.

The evidence from racing lore and history was there. Systematic data, however, was needed in two areas:

Was there some common bond among the large hearted horses of modern times and the storied champions of history? If there was a bond, was it a predictable one?

Before the beginning of modern genetics, horse breeding had been a matter of shrewd guesswork and traditional practices. The guesswork had more often failed to produce champions than it had succeeded. There was agreement that certain traits were inheritable, but it was unclear how they were inherited. The mechanisms of inheritance were unclear.

Before that question could be attacked, however, the more basic question had to be answered:

Was that large heart characteristic truly a contributing factor in performance?

The collection of the data to answer that question began almost by accident.

In 1953, Dr. James D. Steel, a professor and senior lecturer in veterinary medicine at the University of Sydney in Australia, first began using electrocardiography in studies of herbivores (grazing animals). The herbivores he happened to be studying were located mostly in Maurice McCarten's racing stables. McCarten was an Australian racehorse trainer. As Steel's work became more widely known, it was extended to other racing trainers.

Initially, Steel was investigating whether racehorses suffered from heart disease when he noticed an unusual characteristic on the electrocardiogram (ECG) of a leading racehorse of the time, Prince Courtauld.

By using an ECG examination, Steel was able to determine that the heart size of the racehorse was greater than that of a much less successful horse. It was during this time that he coined the term "heart score" to communicate his findings of the heart size on the ECG, which were gained by a correlation of heart weight, stroke volume, cardiac output, and aerobic power.

In doing the ECGs on these two horses, Steel noticed unusually wide QRS complexes in the electrocardiogram of Prince Courtauld. A comparison between this ECG and that of a much less successful three-year-old, Momote, showed a heart score of 130 for Prince Courtauld and a heart score of 86 for Momote.

To summarize the differences in the width of the QRS complex, and to communicate his findings to people who were unfamiliar with ECG terminology, Steel used the term, "heart score" to indicate the mean of the QRS duration recorded from the standard limb leads.

The QRS complex is a series of waves inscribed in the electrocardiogram when the bulk of the heart (ventricles) is electrically activated during each beat. This activation occurs naturally every time the heart beats.

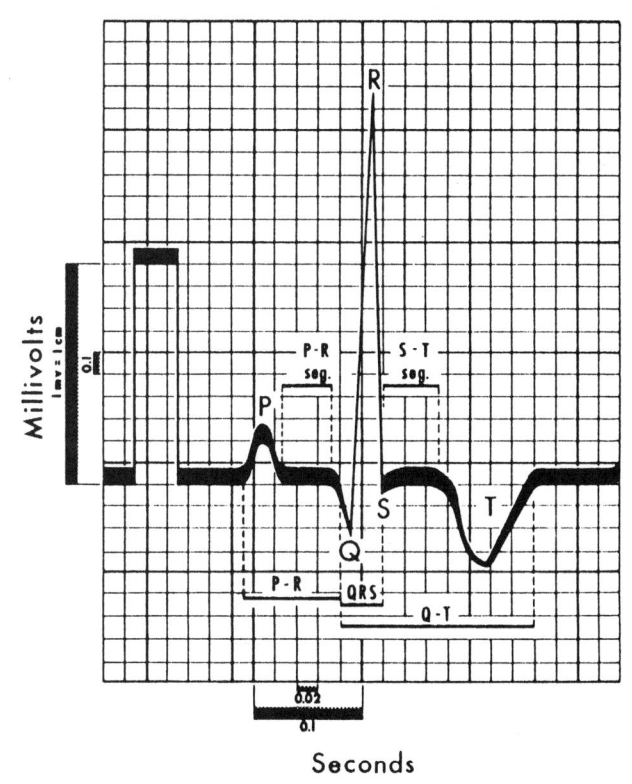

The difference between a small heart and a large heart as shown on the ECG is the width of the QRS wave. The large heart will have a wide QRS baseline. The small heart will show a much narrower baseline.

The ECG is recorded on paper moving at a constant speed. A wider QRS complex represents a longer activation time. The larger the mass (weight of the heart), the longer it takes to activate it and the wider the QRS complex and the bigger the heart score.

This was the critical connection. A wider QRS complex is evidence of a large heart and that large heart can pump more blood with each beat (stroke volume) and therefore per minute (cardiac output).

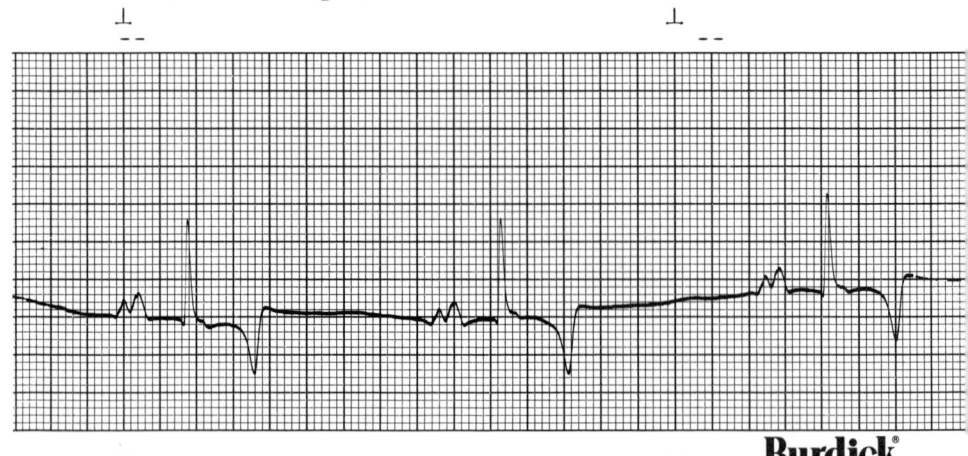

The ECG for Moscow Ballet shows a very wide QRS wave. Moscow Ballet was measured and found to have a heart score of 147

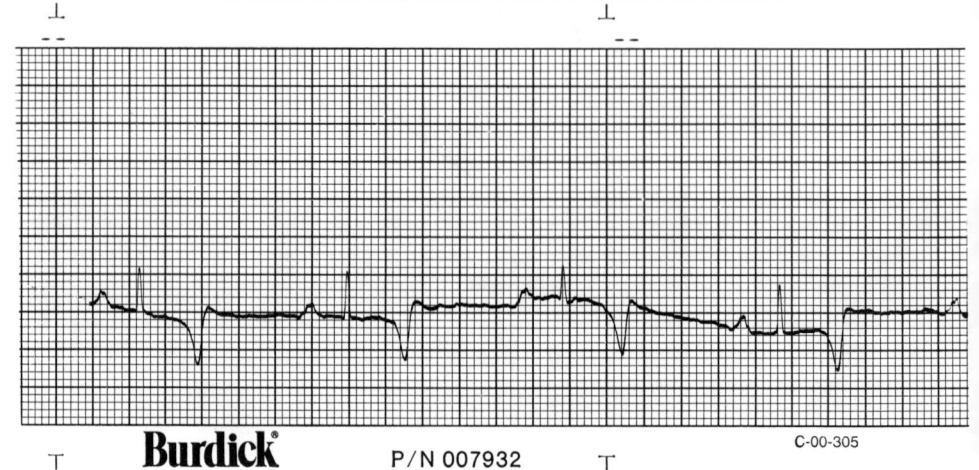

The ECG for horse with a small heart shows a narrow QRS wave.

30

Through his findings, Steel determined that male horses with a heart score of 120 or more were in the large heart category. Fillies and mares with a heart score of 116 or more were in the large heart score category. Horses with heart scores of 103 or less were deemed in the small heart category, and heart scores in between these two categories were considered medium or normal-sized.

Steel's research, therefore, had established a way of determining, non-invasively, the size of a horse's heart.

With this technique available, Steele began to seek a relationship between the heart score and performance. He compiled and studied the racing performance and ECGs of 306 Thoroughbreds. In a preliminary paper in 1957, some of these findings were published. The major part of his work, based on the ECGs of 2,500 Thoroughbreds, was published 6 years later.

Steel had established the crucial link between heart score, heart size and performance. It remained for others to explore that link.

If a link existed between Sham and Secretariat, for instance, the implications would be enormous.

The project which sought to – and did – establish the link is detailed later in this book, but, in brief, it was discovered that both stallions were out of daughters of Princequillo, one of the most successful broodmare sires of 20th century. Because Australian researchers believed the characteristic was sex-linked, which means it was passed along the X chromosome, coming from mother to son to daughter to son and daughter, this was significant.

In addition to leaving a legacy of racing records, Secretariat's most important contribution may well be his great heart which opened the door to the discovery of important clues to a genetic link between large hearts and the X chromosome.

The exploration of that link, however, can best be understood by first exploring some of the work that preceded it.

Chapter 6

The Link Between Heart Score and Performance

In Australia, a growing number of veterinarians studied under Steel and subsequently practiced his brand of equine cardiology. From this group came increasing recognition of the value of heart score in assessing potential for strenuous exercise performance, not only in horse racing, but also in human athletics, greyhound racing, equine endurance riding, and three-day-eventing. For many years in New Zealand, the heart score has been incorporated into the routine cardiology of racehorses.

According to Dr. Anthony Stewart, who studied under Steel and is today one of Australia's leading experts in heart research, the high incidence of large heart scores in successful racehorses suggests that a large heart is a desirable characteristic for racing in the highest class.

In an Australian study of 18 Thoroughbreds, which between them were successful in 22 runnings of either the Victoria Racing Club Victoria Derby (Aust-G1) or the Australian Jockey Club Derby (Aust-G1), it was found that 17 had large heart scores, between 120 and 136, inclusive. In a similar study of 20 winners of either the Caulfield Cup (Aust-G1) or Melbourne Cup (Aust-G1), 15 were found to have heart scores of 120 or more. These were among Australia's most prestigious races.

The heart size indicated in the heart score, Stewart said, appears to contribute approximately 23 percent of the overall quality of the racehorse.

"The heart score provides one easily measured factor among many of significance in the assessment of potential for racing," Stewart said.

According to Stewart, further confirmation of the relationship between the heart score and racing performance has now come from workers independent of the groups in Australia and New Zealand.

"From Denmark, Nielsen and Vibe-Petersen reported highly significant correlations between heart score and both kilometre time and stakes money won by trotting horses," Stewart said. "Guarded support has also come from Physick-Sheard and Hendren, studying Standardbreds in Canada.

"In the United Kingdom, Leadon, Cunningham, Mahon and Todd reported a significant correlation between heart score and Timeform ratings in 71 3-year-olds, but not in 70 2-year-olds, yet strangely, both correlation coefficients (r-0.359 and 0.320 respectively) statistically seemed to be highly significant."

Stewart said not all groups have been successful in detecting a relationship between heart score and racing performance. He cites a study done in the United States by Gross, Muir, Pipers, and Hamlin which recognized no correlation. Stewart points out, though, that the study comprised only 12 Thoroughbreds, the heart scores of which had been obtained when the animals were yearlings.

As the heart in a horse grows until he is three years of age, Stewart said, anyone attempting to use the measurement of a heart in a yearling, is merely guessing at what the size might eventually be.

In addition to Thoroughbreds, Australian researchers and other groups abroad have studied Standardbreds as well and have documented the same relationship between large hearts and high heart scores to performance as was found in the Thoroughbred.

According to Stewart, a group of researchers in Australia did a study on families of Standardbreds in the 1960s. Stewart said the researchers felt from what they discovered with measurements of the horses that the characteristic appeared to be a sex-linked co-dominant genetic trait on the X chromosome. They found the heart size of the female offspring were either the sire's or the dam's or a blending of the two with the colt's heart size coming from the dam.

The large heart characteristic is felt to be just as valuable in a trotting horse as in a flat-racing animal.

In the study of 195 trotting horses by Nielsen and Vibe-Petersen in Denmark, they reported a mean correlation coefficient between kilometer time and heart score of 0.47. Using the correlation between the heart score and the performance parameter, highest standard of race won by the horse, the figure indicates that 22 percent of the performance parameter can be attributed to the heart score.

These estimates put the heart score theory in reasonable context against other factors contributing to the performance and quality of the racehorse.

"The estimates of 22-23 percent still leave approximately 77 percent of the quality to be derived from other factors, as many of which as possible should be taken into account when assessing the animal," Stewart said. "Yet amongst all these variables, for one easily-measured factor, the heart score, to account for 23 percent provides a useful contribution to the overall assessment of potential for racing."

In the British study done by Leadon, Cunningham, Mahon, and Todd, Stewart said, it was noted that horses grouped according to heart score showed an increasing minimum Timeform rating with each increment in heart score; i.e., as the heart score rose, a higher minimum performance was achieved within the group of horses with that heart score.

"In an individual horse with a high heart score there is a danger that this may engender unrealistically high expectations, unless one takes into account the many other factors contributing to the quality and performance of the racehorse," Stewart said. "Of more practical use may be the fact that horses with lower heart scores do not perform as well or consistently in high class racing as do horses with high heart scores, and a guarded prognosis should be made when the heart score is medium-low."

The incidence of large heart scores is approximately 25 percent in the overall racehorse population, Stewart said.

"If a high heart score is an important characteristic for performance, its incidence among successful horses should be substantially higher," he said, adding that this effect has been shown to be present in several studies, including those done with the Victoria Derby, AJC Derby, Melbourne Cup, and Caulfield Cup.

"In studying elite trotters competing in the 1979 International race, the Copenhagen Cup, Nielsen and Vibe-Petersen found large heart scores of 124 or higher in all eight runners," Stewart said. "This incidence of 100 percent large heart scores contrasted with an incidence of 28 percent (heart score of 117 or higher) among 175 mares and stallions in the general population studied by these workers, and their mean heart score for mature mares and stallions of 110.4, with a standard deviation of 12.8.

"In Standardbreds, Steel too had noted the occurrence of consistently high heart scores in the horses contesting the 1960 Yonkers International Pacing Series in New York, and also in better performed pacers here at Harold Park."

In Australia, they did a retrospective study of Thoroughbreds. The weight-for-age races during the Spring Racing Carnival in Melbourne, were taken as representative of Australian racing of the highest class. According to Stewart, in this study 35 weight-for-age winners with recorded heart scores were identified, and 31 of these had heart scores between 120 and 140 inclusive. The other four had heart scores of 113.

"Thus 89 percent of this population of high-class winners had large heart scores," he said.

From these statistics, Stewart said, again it may be concluded that large heart scores are a desirable characteristic for racing in the highest class. But, he cautioned, never forget the horse with the normal sized heart, who is so superbly endowed with other characteristics to overcome any advantage lost from a smaller heart.

"From the statistics, however, in an industry so orientated toward odds, one may conclude that in high-class racing the chances of success for a horse with a low heart score are correspondingly lower," he said.

Steel and Stewart have reported results from studies demonstrating a relationship between high heart score and heart weight. In their studies, they reported heart scores of individual horses, varying from 86 to 146, with heart weights from 1.9 kg (4.18 pounds) to 6.1 kg (13.42 pounds), and a highly significant correlation between heart score and heart weight.

Famous Racehorses' Heart Weights & Scores

Name of Horse (color, sex, year of birth)	Heart Weight	Heart Score
Eclipse (ch.h. 1764)	14 lbs	
Phar Lap (ch.g. 1926)	14 lbs	
Secretariat (ch.h. 1970)	22 lbs	
Sham (ch.h. 1970)	18 lbs*	
Star Kingdom (ch.h 1946)	14 lbs	
Mill Reef (b.h. 1968)	16.94 lbs*	
Easy Goer (ch.h. 1986)	15 lbs	
Althea (ch.m. 1981)	15 lbs	
Hyperion (ch.h. 1930)		133
Moscow Ballet (b.h. 1982)		147
Soviet Problem (ch.m. 1990)		150
The Last Red (ch.m. 1993-twin)		140
Desert Secret (IRE) (b.h. 1990)		140
Key To The Mint (b.h. 1969)	15.8 lbs	157
Northern Dancer (b.h. 1961)		150
Killaloe (b.m. 1970)	12.9 lbs	
Tulloch (AUS)(b.h. 1954)	13.5 lbs	136
Manikato (AUS)(ch.g. 1975)		123
Kingston Town (AUS) (blk.g. 1976)		130
Vo Rogue (b.g. 1983)		130

Note: Pathological enlargement found in the hearts during autopsy can add two to three pounds or more to the heart weight.
* *Some pathological enlargement*

According to a study conducted by Australian scientists comparing heart score to heart weight at autopsy, the following table was established.

Comparing Heart Score and Heart Weight

Heart Score	Heart Weight
100	6.6 lbs
110	7.36 lbs
120	10.12 lbs
130	11.88 lbs
140	13.64 lbs
150	15.4 lbs
160	17.16 lbs

Chapter 7

The 120 Heart Score Advantage

To be useful to horse breeders, heart size must be quantified.

In 1963, Steel reported a highly significant correlation between the QRS duration and the heart weight at autopsy in 34 racehorses (r32= + 0.89, P <0.001). By 1970 the number of autopsies studied in the relationship between heart score and heart weight had increased to 55, with a slight increase in the correlation coefficient (r53 = 0.92, P< 0.001).

From these studies, they were able to establish a table of averages relating heart score to heart weight. In this table, a heart score of 100 is equal to a weight of 3.0 kg. One kg is equal to 2.2 pounds, so a 100 heart score would relate to a 6.6 pound heart. A heart score of 110 is 3.8 kg (7.36 pounds), 120 is 4.6 kg (10.12 pounds), 130 is 5.4 kg (11.88 pounds), 140 is 6.2 kg (13.64 pounds), 150 is 7 kg (15.4 pounds), 160 is 7.8 kg (17.16 pounds).

Heart Score, Heart Weight and Stroke Volume

Heart Score (msec.)	Heart Weight (kg)**	Stroke Volume (litres)	Cardiac Output (L/min. at max exercise)#
100	3.0	0.5	100
110	3.8	0.75	150
120	4.6	1.0	200
130	5.4	1.25	250

*Estimated by Steel (Unpublished data, 1977) ** kg.=2.2 lbs.
#Assuming a heart rate of 200 beats per minute

Mill Reef, when he died, had a heart that weighed 7.7 kg (16.94 pounds). Based on the Australian scale, that would give him a heart score of approximately 158. Based on this scale, Secretariat's heart score could be estimated at approximately 180. Sham, whose heart weighed 18 pounds at autopsy, but who had some pathological enlargement, would probably be in the 150 range on heart score.

In the Australian table, the mean heart score was 111.5 plus or minus 1.45 msec (points in a heart score). The mean heart weight was 3.92 kg (8.6 pounds) plus or minus 0.104 kg (.23 pounds).

According to Stewart, from these studies they concluded that individual heart scores of 120 or more represent hearts that are larger than average and heart scores of 103 or less represent hearts smaller than average.

Stewart said these averages may be modified slightly to take sex difference into account. The mean heart scores of fillies and mares are approximately 4 msec. less than those of male horses. Thus in fillies and mares, a heart score of 116 or more is taken as representing large hearts.

The relationships between heart scores and heart weight in the racehorse support the conclusion drawn by Wilson and Herman in 1930 that the "QRS interval is an accurate measure of the time required for the ventricular muscle to pass into the active state." As a result, it can be concluded that a longer QRS duration indicates a larger mass of ventricular muscle.

This has been demonstrated in other species as well. The significant relationships of the heart score to cardiac transverse diameter in Olympic athletes and to heart weight in greyhounds have confirmed the value of heart score as an indicator of heart size. Studies correlating the heart score and aerobic power of high class athletes further suggested a relationship between these two estimates, Stewart said, perhaps through a common relationship to cardiac output.

Steel, shortly before his death, visited the Japan Racing Association Equine Health Laboratory where he undertook some preliminary studies regarding cardiac output and heart score in horses. According to Stewart, these early observations led Steel to estimate a relationship between stroke volume, heart weight, and heart score in the horses he studied, which led to the table relating heart score to heart weight.

In addition to those two factors, Steel also measured the stroke volume and cardiac output of horses at maximum exercise (assuming a heart rate of 200 beats per minute).

The difference in heart score between 100 and 120 may be reflecting much greater differences in cardiac function, in terms of stroke volume and cardiac output than might have been expected from an apparent difference in heart score of 20 percent.

Hence, in a functional sense, Stewart said, "One should expect very different exercise performance from the horse with the large heart, with an estimated stroke volume of a liter or more, compared with the horse with a small heart, estimated to pump only half a liter or so."

To keep the information gleaned in terms of heart score and racing performance in perspective of the galloping horse, one must consider the metabolic demands of the skeletal muscles. The racehorse, unlike the human athlete, has skeletal muscle fibers with high oxidative metabolism for both sprinting and staying.

"Thus a high cardiac output during exercise represents an enormous advantage to the racehorse with the large heart, whether it be for speed or stamina," Stewart said. "It may now be concluded that the relationship between heart score and stroke volume, the high heart rate during racing, and the large oxygen requirements of the horse galloping, provide a sound physiological basis for the relationships between the heart score and racing performance in all distances over which the Thoroughbred races."

The large heart has been a consistent characteristic found in the very top racehorses.

"That is one of the reasons we are conducting this study," said equine cardiologist Dr. Frederick Fregin, Director of the Marion duPont Scott Equine Medical Center at Virginia Tech in Leesburg, Va. "You don't usually find small hearts in the best runners.

"We've measured more than 120 horses now and the evidence has been very consistent. Dr. Steel and Dr. Stewart have shown significant correlation between heart score and racing performance in their research that indicated that a large heart was at least one factor that could be associated with a successful racehorse.

"We started on this trail more than 40 years ago. Now maybe we can finally put it all together and see where it starts. We have long been selecting horses and breeding horses because of their racing performance and what we may have actually been doing has been to unknowingly select and breed animals with large hearts."

There have been notable exceptions like Bold Ruler and Caro, who were found to have normal sized hearts at autopsy. There will always be individuals who have such superb characteristics in other areas as to make up for smaller hearts.

Chapter 8

Trotters & Heart Score

In first looking at racehorses with large heart scores, the Australians had seen a pattern of performance. This pattern indicated that horses with large hearts performed more successfully and consistently in the top class races than horses with small hearts. Because of this observation, studies were conducted involving both flat-racers and trotters, not only in Australia, but abroad as well.

In the Denmark study of trotters by Nielsen and Vibe-Petersen, of the Royal Veterinary and Agricultural University in Copenhagen, it was observed that there was a positive correlation between heart scores and earnings in races. The two Danish researchers recorded ECGs on 230 horses in training at Charlottenlund Trotting Track near Copenhagen, Denmark.

According to their 1980 report of the study, on 11 horses recordings were made in two (seven horses) and three (four horses) consecutive years. Additional recordings were made in May 1970, of eight horses starting in the international race, the Copenhagen Cup.

Care was taken to insure that the ECGs were recorded while the horse was either standing relaxed in its stall or in a field. The horses were posed to be standing with an even distribution on all four limbs with the left forefoot slightly in front of the right foot. Using silver-plated electrodes, which were applied just distal to the elbow and stifle joints by means of rubber straps and the standard limb leads plus three augmented voltage leads, the ECG was recorded using the method developed by Dr. James Steel and Dr. Anthony Stewart of Australia.

Nielsen and Vibe-Petersen did not collect information on the racing performance of the horses until after all the ECG recordings had been processed.

After collecting the racing performance data from the Danish Trotting Society, all the information, including the best kilometer time and the earnings, was fed into a computer for a statistical analysis.

In their study, Nielsen and Vibe-Petersen reported that heart scores increased with age and training. Yearlings were reported to have an average heart score of 90 which increased to 110 by the age of five. They found a highly significant correlation between heart score and kilometer time in horses 4 years old and older, when the heart was fully grown. The level of significance was less in younger horses.

Heart Scores in Mares and Stallions of Different Age

Age	#	Mare Heart Score	SD*	#	Stallion Heart Score	SD*	#	Total Heart Score	SD*
1	4	90	nd**	4	93	nd**	8	91.3	13.8
2	19	92.9	12.1	33	99.5	9.2	52	97.1	10.7
3	26	98.4	11.7	37	107.8	12.6	63	103.9	13.0
4	17	97.7	12.4	34	108.4	11.9	51	104.8	13.0
>5	21	107.2	13.7	50	111.7	12.2	71	110.4	12.8

*SD = Standard Deviation   **nd = not done
(reprinted from the Equine Veterinary Journal 12 (2) 81-84)

They found a positive correlation between earnings in races and heart scores. Horses with heart scores above 115 earned considerably more than horses with heart scores below this figure. The relationship was closer in stallions than in mares.

Heart Scores and Racing Performance in Stallions and Mares

Heart score	Number horses	Average starts per horse	Average stakes per horse(DKr)*	Average stakes per start (DKr)
Stallions				
< 95	18	11	8,115	706
96-105	31	17	14,722	1,216
106-115	32	19	24,125	1,623
116-125	33	20	31,665	1,610
126-135	8	21	65,050	3,237
Mares				
< 95	17	18	21,215	1,360
96-105	17	20	13,756	854
106-115	11	19	29,277	1,511
116-125	7	19	29,043	1,552
126-135	1	42	79,120	1,884

*Danish Kroner
(reprinted from the Equine Veterinary Journal 12 (2) 81-84)

In terms of earning power, the 41 stallions with heart scores above 115 earned more than double what the 81 stallions with heart scores below 115 earned.

The relationship was not as well defined in the group of mares studied. Mares with heart scores below 95 raced rather well compared to mares with higher heart scores. But, the small group of eight mares which had heart scores exceeding 115 had average stakes earnings that were considerably higher than the 45 mares with lower heart scores.

In the study of the eight elite international trotting horses competing in the 1979 Copenhagen Cup, the heart scores ranged from 124 to 152, which was considerably higher than the level recorded in the other horses that Nielsen and Vibe-Petersen found at a local trotting track in Copenhagen, which they used for their study. Several of the horses competing in the Copenhagen Cup were ranked among the world's best trotters.

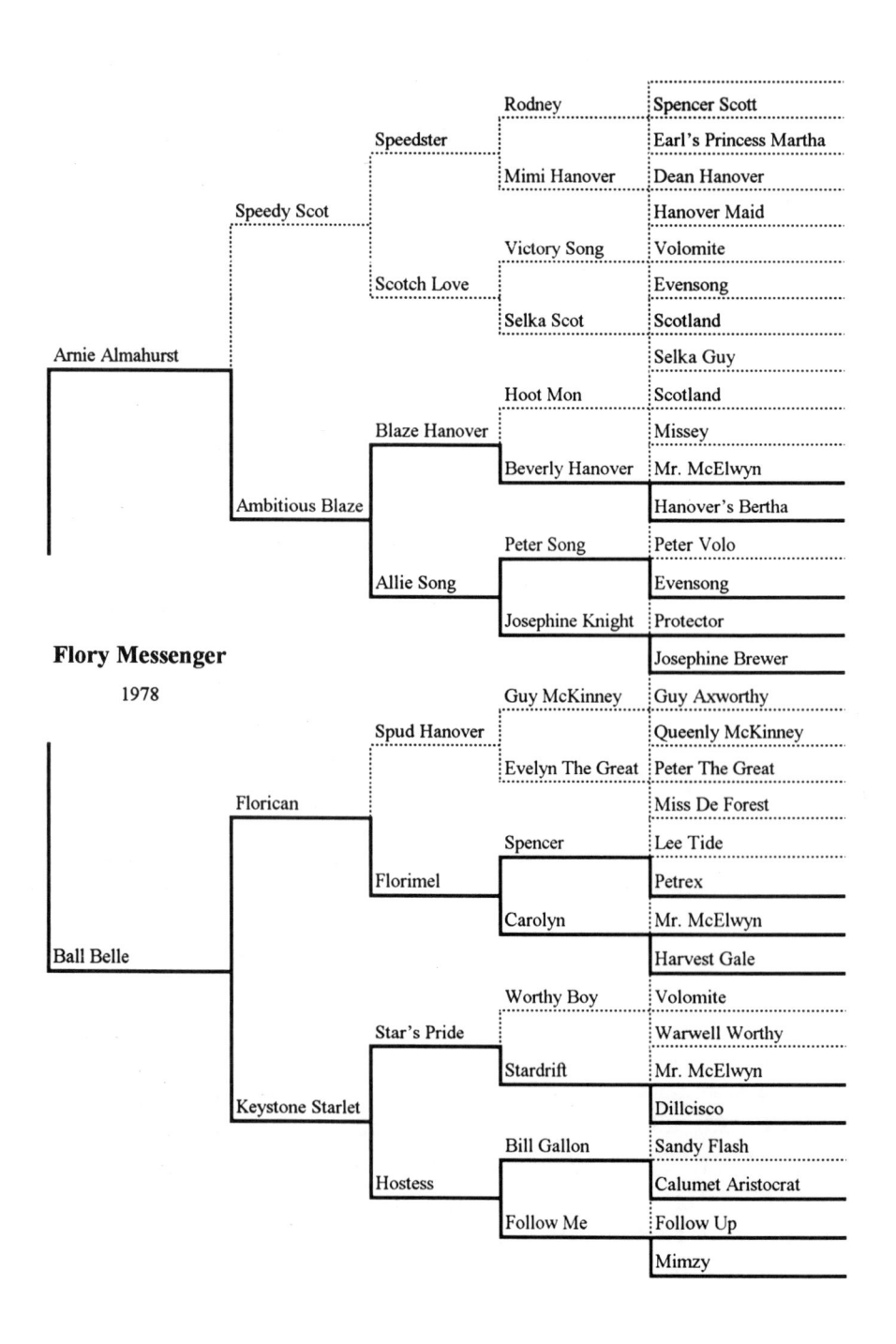

Flory Messenger
1978

- Arnie Almahurst
  - Speedy Scot
    - Speedster
      - Rodney
        - Spencer Scott
        - Earl's Princess Martha
      - Mimi Hanover
        - Dean Hanover
        - Hanover Maid
    - Scotch Love
      - Victory Song
        - Volomite
        - Evensong
      - Selka Scot
        - Scotland
        - Selka Guy
  - Ambitious Blaze
    - Blaze Hanover
      - Hoot Mon
        - Scotland
        - Missey
      - Beverly Hanover
        - Mr. McElwyn
        - Hanover's Bertha
    - Allie Song
      - Peter Song
        - Peter Volo
        - Evensong
      - Josephine Knight
        - Protector
        - Josephine Brewer

- Ball Belle
  - Florican
    - Spud Hanover
      - Guy McKinney
        - Guy Axworthy
        - Queenly McKinney
      - Evelyn The Great
        - Peter The Great
        - Miss De Forest
    - Florimel
      - Spencer
        - Lee Tide
        - Petrex
      - Carolyn
        - Mr. McElwyn
        - Harvest Gale
  - Keystone Starlet
    - Star's Pride
      - Worthy Boy
        - Volomite
        - Warwell Worthy
      - Stardrift
        - Mr. McElwyn
        - Dillcisco
    - Hostess
      - Bill Gallon
        - Sandy Flash
        - Calumet Aristocrat
      - Follow Me
        - Follow Up
        - Mimzy

In the summary of their findings, Nielsen and Vibe-Petersen concluded that heart score is correlated with heart weight and is determined by a combination of heredity, age, growth, and by intensity of physical training. Their study confirmed and extended the data on heart score presented by Steel and his colleagues.

According to the report, "The results imply that a horse with a high heart score, i.e., a large ventricular myocardium, possesses a cardiac reserve of crucial importance for its qualities as a race horse.

"This may be due to greater myocardial strength and contractibility and to a greater distolic filling volume, resulting in a larger stroke volume. Bergsten (1974) measured minute volumes of 100 to 175 litres in horses trotting at submaximal speed on a tread mill. The cardiac output of a trotter racing at full speed is not known but it seems rather likely that a horse with a larger myocardial mass has an advantage over horses with a smaller cardiac reserve."

The researchers concluded that heart score appears to be a useful and simple indicator of racing potential in a trotting horse. They suggested it could be used as a screening device in young horses starting in training.

A study, measuring two producing Standardbred mares at Castleton Farm in Lexington, KY, found two large hearts. The largest heart was found in Flory Messenger, who had a heart score of 140. As a trotter, Flory Messenger, by Arnie Almahurst out of Ball Belle by Florican, had earned $35,484 at three.

Foaled in 1978, Flory Messenger has produced 13 foals. The best, so far, has been her first, a 1983 colt, Express Ride, by Super Bowl, who earned more than $1 million. Because he was a colt, it is certain that he was trotting with Flory Messenger's heart. She also produced the sire, Carry The Message, by Royal Prestige, who earned $206,011.

It is interesting to note that on the X chromosome line on the bottom of Flory Messenger's pedigree, is the sire Star's

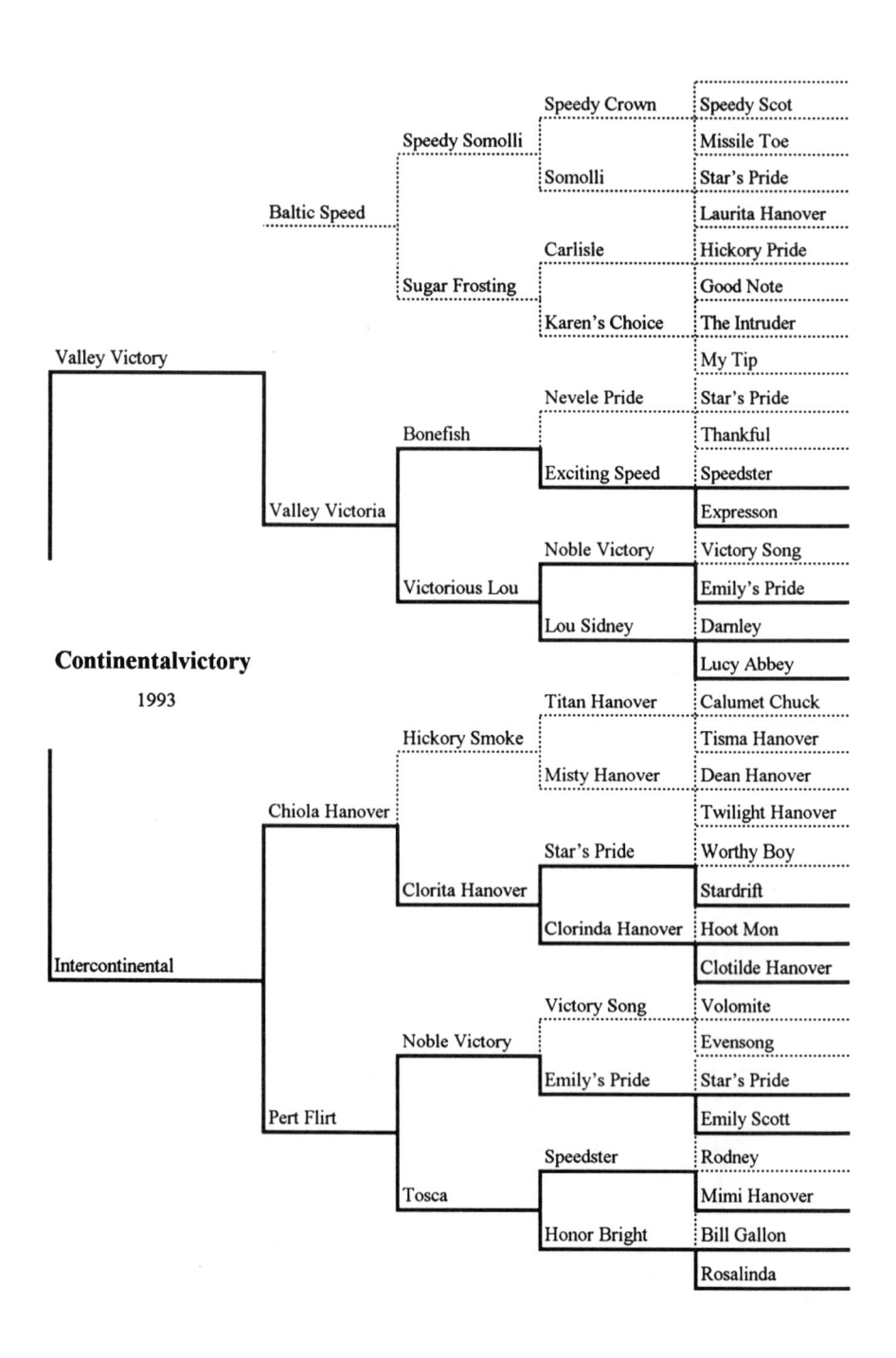

Continentalvictory
1993

Valley Victory
- Baltic Speed
  - Speedy Somolli
    - Speedy Crown
      - Speedy Scot
      - Missile Toe
    - Somolli
      - Star's Pride
      - Laurita Hanover
  - Sugar Frosting
    - Carlisle
      - Hickory Pride
      - Good Note
    - Karen's Choice
      - The Intruder
      - My Tip
- Valley Victoria
  - Bonefish
    - Nevele Pride
      - Star's Pride
      - Thankful
    - Exciting Speed
      - Speedster
      - Expresson
  - Victorious Lou
    - Noble Victory
      - Victory Song
      - Emily's Pride
    - Lou Sidney
      - Darnley
      - Lucy Abbey

Intercontinental
- Chiola Hanover
  - Hickory Smoke
    - Titan Hanover
      - Calumet Chuck
      - Tisma Hanover
    - Misty Hanover
      - Dean Hanover
      - Twilight Hanover
  - Clorita Hanover
    - Star's Pride
      - Worthy Boy
      - Stardrift
    - Clorinda Hanover
      - Hoot Mon
      - Clotilde Hanover
- Pert Flirt
  - Noble Victory
    - Victory Song
      - Volomite
      - Evensong
    - Emily's Pride
      - Star's Pride
      - Emily Scott
  - Tosca
    - Speedster
      - Rodney
      - Mimi Hanover
    - Honor Bright
      - Bill Gallon
      - Rosalinda

Pride, who seems, based on the pattern of performance, the most likely source of her large heart.

In the pedigree of the outstanding trotting filly, Continentalvictory, who won the 1996 Hambletonian, she has Star's Pride on three of her heart lines. Star's Pride is on the bottom of her sire, Valley Victory's pedigree, and on the bottom of her broodmare sire, Chiola Hanover's pedigree, as well as on the bottom of her maternal granddam, Pert Flirt's sire's pedigree.

Both the top and bottom of Continentalvictory's pedigree heart lines contain the sire, Noble Victory, whose dam, Emily's Pride is a daughter of Star's Pride. This makes it very likely that the heart she carries came from Star's Pride.

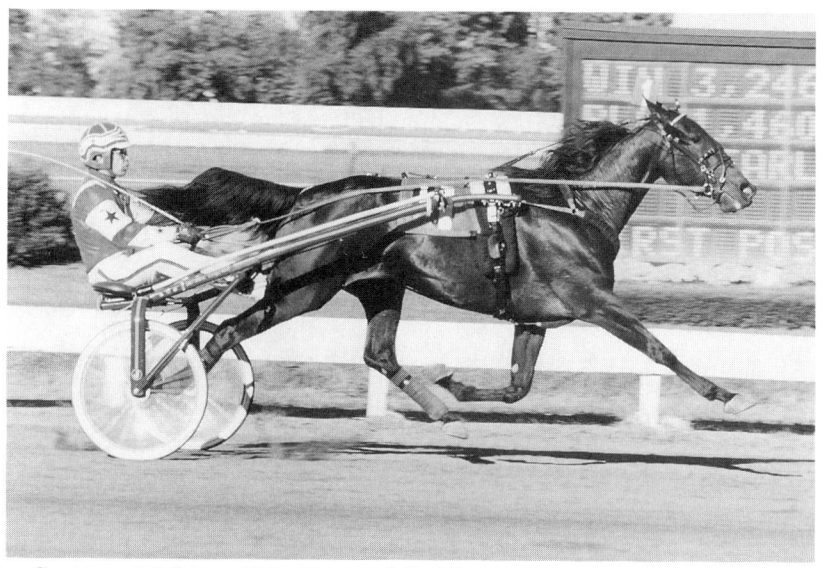

Continentalvictory 1996 Horse of the Year and Hambletonian winner
(Photo by Monica Thors)

The other mare, Tarport Cheer, who had a heart score of 133, had zero earnings, but has produced a number of outstanding foals, including the Tarport Hap, by Most Happy Fella, who earned $688,664; Tyler B, by Most Happy Fella, who earned $687,388; and Cheery Hello, by Albatross, who

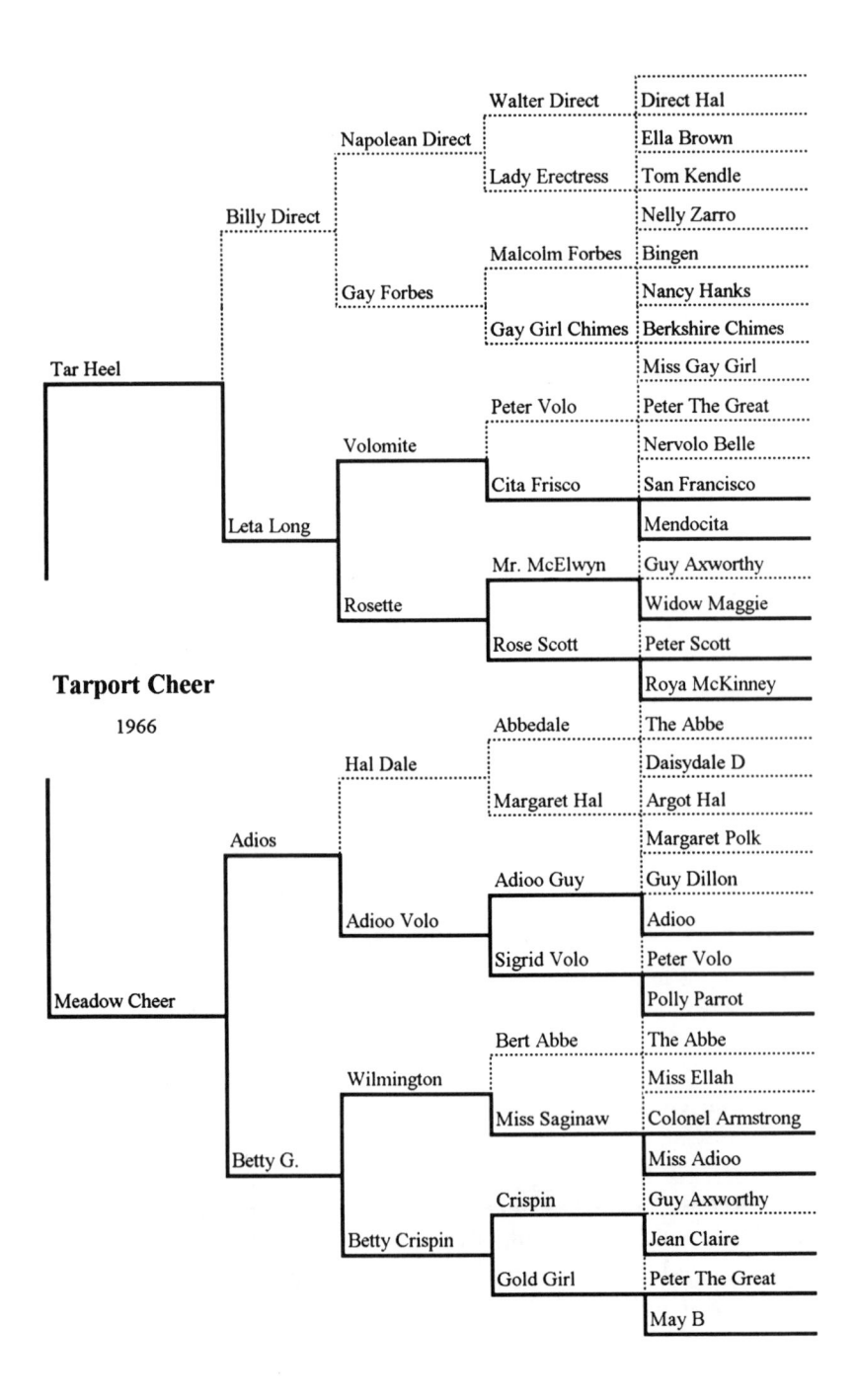

Tarport Cheer

1966

Tar Heel

- Billy Direct
  - Napolean Direct
    - Walter Direct
      - Direct Hal
      - Ella Brown
    - Lady Erectress
      - Tom Kendle
      - Nelly Zarro
  - Gay Forbes
    - Malcolm Forbes
      - Bingen
      - Nancy Hanks
    - Gay Girl Chimes
      - Berkshire Chimes
      - Miss Gay Girl
- Leta Long
  - Volomite
    - Peter Volo
      - Peter The Great
      - Nervolo Belle
    - Cita Frisco
      - San Francisco
      - Mendocita
  - Rosette
    - Mr. McElwyn
      - Guy Axworthy
      - Widow Maggie
    - Rose Scott
      - Peter Scott
      - Roya McKinney

Meadow Cheer

- Adios
  - Hal Dale
    - Abbedale
      - The Abbe
      - Daisydale D
    - Margaret Hal
      - Argot Hal
      - Margaret Polk
  - Adioo Volo
    - Adioo Guy
      - Guy Dillon
      - Adioo
    - Sigrid Volo
      - Peter Volo
      - Polly Parrot
- Betty G.
  - Wilmington
    - Bert Abbe
      - The Abbe
      - Miss Ellah
    - Miss Saginaw
      - Colonel Armstrong
      - Miss Adioo
  - Betty Crispin
    - Crispin
      - Guy Axworthy
      - Jean Claire
    - Gold Girl
      - Peter The Great
      - May B

earned $869,619.

Foaled in 1966, Tarport Cheer, now retired, has produced 16 foals. Her pedigree is more difficult to trace for heart sized patterns of performance, since many of the dams are unraced, but Tarport Cheer's heart may have come from Volomite, the sire of Letalong, the dam of her sire, Tar Heel.

Peace Corps, widely held as the greatest trotting mare of all time with earnings of more than $4.9 million, shares the large heart lines found in Continentalvictory's pedigree, as well as those of Valley Victory, Tarport Cheer and Flory Messenger.

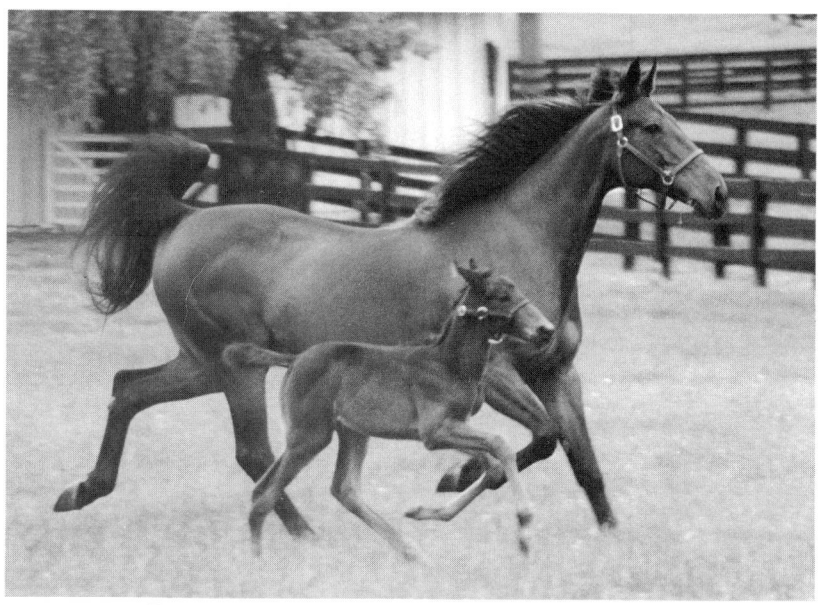

Peace Corps with her first foal (by Mack Lobell)
Photo by Marianna Haun

Through her sire, Baltic Speed, she has the heart line to Volomite through her maternal granddam, Karen's Choice. Volomite is the large heart line found in Tarport Cheer's pedigree, an outstanding broodmare that had a heart score of 133.

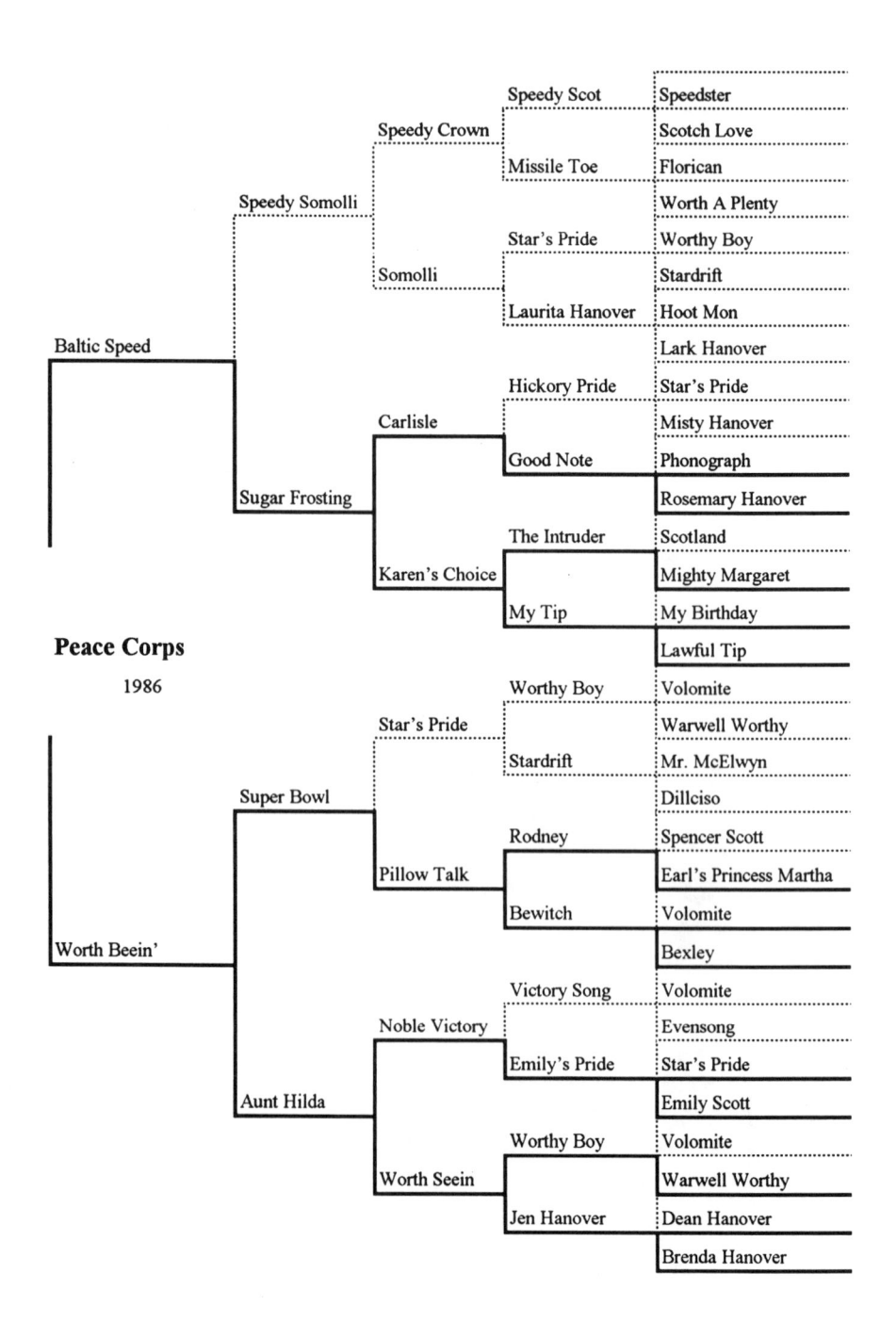

Peace Corps
1986

Baltic Speed
- Speedy Somolli
  - Speedy Crown
    - Speedy Scot
      - Speedster
      - Scotch Love
    - Missile Toe
      - Florican
      - Worth A Plenty
  - Somolli
    - Star's Pride
      - Worthy Boy
      - Stardrift
    - Laurita Hanover
      - Hoot Mon
      - Lark Hanover
- Sugar Frosting
  - Carlisle
    - Hickory Pride
      - Star's Pride
      - Misty Hanover
    - Good Note
      - Phonograph
      - Rosemary Hanover
  - Karen's Choice
    - The Intruder
      - Scotland
      - Mighty Margaret
    - My Tip
      - My Birthday
      - Lawful Tip

Worth Beein'
- Super Bowl
  - Star's Pride
    - Worthy Boy
      - Volomite
      - Warwell Worthy
    - Stardrift
      - Mr. McElwyn
      - Dillciso
  - Pillow Talk
    - Rodney
      - Spencer Scott
      - Earl's Princess Martha
    - Bewitch
      - Volomite
      - Bexley
- Aunt Hilda
  - Noble Victory
    - Victory Song
      - Volomite
      - Evensong
    - Emily's Pride
      - Star's Pride
      - Emily Scott
  - Worth Seein
    - Worthy Boy
      - Volomite
      - Warwell Worthy
    - Jen Hanover
      - Dean Hanover
      - Brenda Hanover

The most impressive heart lines in Peace Corps' pedigree are found on her bottom side, through her dam, Worth Beein'. On the bottom side of the pedigree of her broodmare sire Super Bowl, Peace Corps tracks to Volomite through his daughter, Bewitch. But the most interesting heart line in her pedigree is that of her maternal granddam, Aunt Hilda, a daughter of Noble Victory out of Emily's Pride. This Star's Pride line is one she shares with trotting sensation, Continentalvictory, who goes through Emily's Pride to Star's Pride through her sire, Valley Victory, and her dam, Intercontinental.

Flory Messenger, who had a heart score of 140, also tracks to Star's Pride through her granddam, Keystone Starlet.

By now, the evidence is overwhelming that heart size, heart score and performance are linked.

The historical and biological questions have been answered.

They leave, though the most important question:

Is heart size predictably inheritable?

That is the genetic question.

PART III

THE GENETIC SEARCH

Chapter 9

Searching for the Heart Score Genes

It was absolutely clear by now that heart score and heart size were vitally important in the makeup of a great champion.

That information was of great biological importance. It did not, however, help with the most important question:

Were great hearts predictably inheritable?

The answer to that question lies in the interplay of historical knowledge of the great horses, the collection of heart size data of present-day champions and the modern study of genetics.

That firmly established correlation between heart score and performance led to the full-scale attempt by researchers to find out if heart size and heart score were inheritable.

In their studies of this factor, the Australians first noted the possibility of sex linkage in the inheritance of the large heart in the Thoroughbreds. Stewart estimated the heritability of the heart score is 38 percent.

Genetically, the mare has two X chromosomes – one she gets from her sire and one she gets from her dam. The stallion has one X chromosome, which he receives from his dam and gives to his daughters, and one Y chromosome which he gets from his sire and gives to his sons. Because the large heart characteristic passes on the X chromosome, the sire cannot give it to his sons, only to his daughters.

In order for a colt to inherit the large heart, he must receive it from his dam. A filly can receive it from either the sire or the dam, depending upon which X is dominant. In

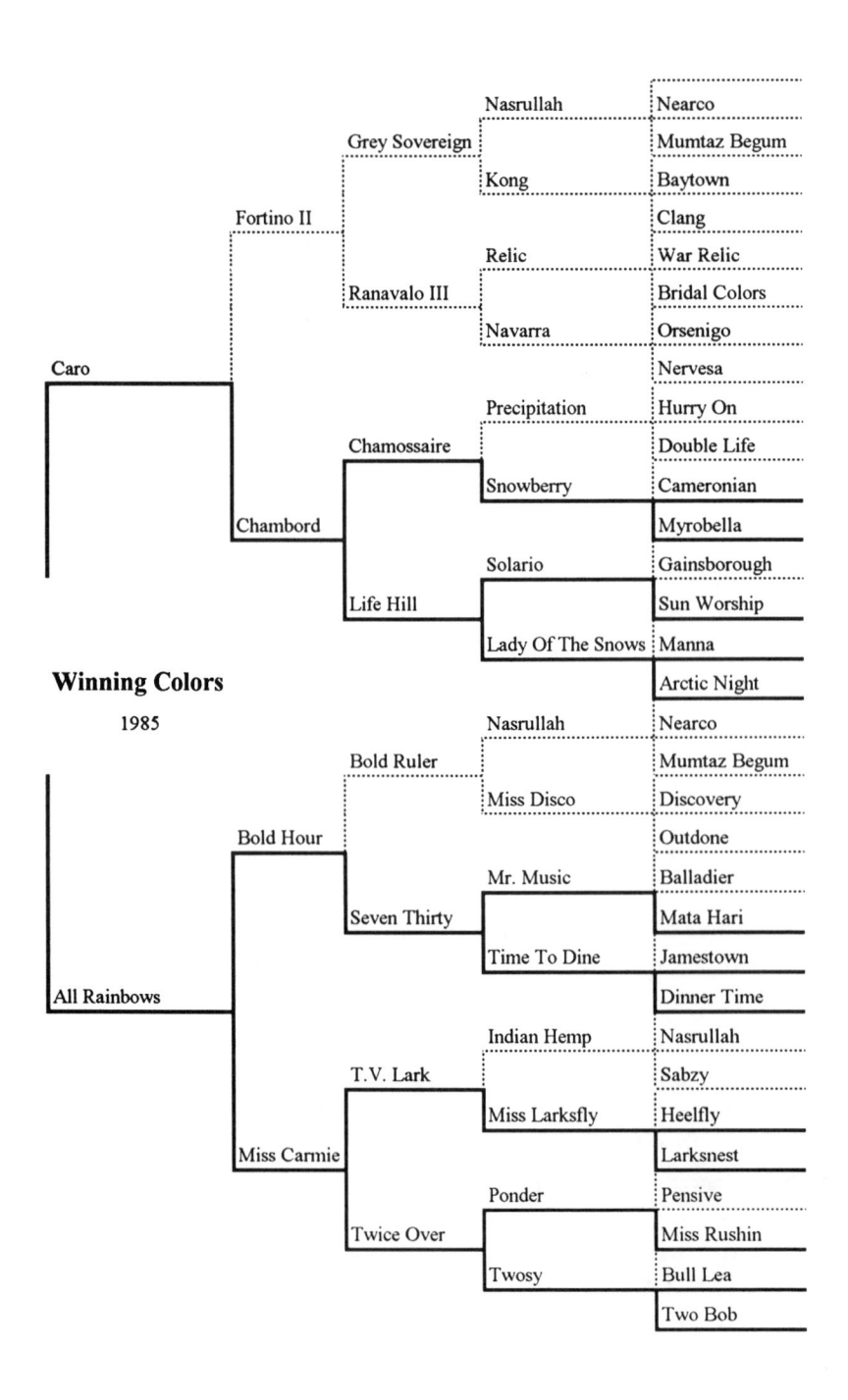

Winning Colors
1985

Caro
- Fortino II
  - Grey Sovereign
    - Nasrullah
      - Nearco
      - Mumtaz Begum
    - Kong
      - Baytown
      - Clang
  - Ranavalo III
    - Relic
      - War Relic
      - Bridal Colors
    - Navarra
      - Orsenigo
      - Nervesa
- Chambord
  - Chamossaire
    - Precipitation
      - Hurry On
      - Double Life
    - Snowberry
      - Cameronian
      - Myrobella
  - Life Hill
    - Solario
      - Gainsborough
      - Sun Worship
    - Lady Of The Snows
      - Manna
      - Arctic Night

All Rainbows
- Bold Hour
  - Bold Ruler
    - Nasrullah
      - Nearco
      - Mumtaz Begum
    - Miss Disco
      - Discovery
      - Outdone
  - Seven Thirty
    - Mr. Music
      - Balladier
      - Mata Hari
    - Time To Dine
      - Jamestown
      - Dinner Time
- Miss Carmie
  - T.V. Lark
    - Indian Hemp
      - Nasrullah
      - Sabzy
    - Miss Larksfly
      - Heelfly
      - Larksnest
  - Twice Over
    - Ponder
      - Pensive
      - Miss Rushin
    - Twosy
      - Bull Lea
      - Two Bob

ongoing studies measuring horses for this characteristic, it appears that when the subject is a filly, she has a 50-50 chance of receiving the heart of either her sire or her dam.

One famous example of a champion filly receiving her dam's heart is Winning Colors, winner of the 1988 Kentucky Derby. Winning Colors, who has a large heart, was by the French champion Caro. Her sire was discovered to have a normal-sized heart during his autopsy, performed by Swerczek the day after he did the autopsy on Secretariat in 1989. Swerczek said Caro's heart seemed very small, but that was probably in comparison to Secretariat's huge heart.

"It was actually a normal-sized heart," Swerczek said, who did not weigh Caro's heart.

Winning Color's large heart probably came up the tail female line of her pedigree. Her dam, All Rainbows, was by Bold Hour out of Miss Carmie, who had outstanding large heart lines on all of her X chromosome lines.

"In our studies, dams have been shown to have greater influence than sires on the heart score of their progeny," Stewart said. "Sires have a greater influence on their daughters' heart scores than on their sons. Thus, we feel the inheritance of heart size in the racehorse is sex-linked."

Sex linkage would affect the regression coefficients because the dam, who has two X chromosomes, passes an X chromosome to both sexes of her progeny. The sire has one X chromosome, which he gets from his dam and passes to his daughter, and one Y chromosome, which he gets from his sire and passes to his son. If the characteristic is on the X chromosome, then the sire cannot pass it on to his son. The son can only receive it from his dam. The filly, with two X chromosomes, can receive the characteristic from either her sire or her dam, depending upon which X is dominant.

These facts, combined with the traditional approach to breeding which had emphasized the sire and almost ignored the dam, had led to the frustrating inability of breeders to produce a consistent line of champions.

Genetic Pedigree

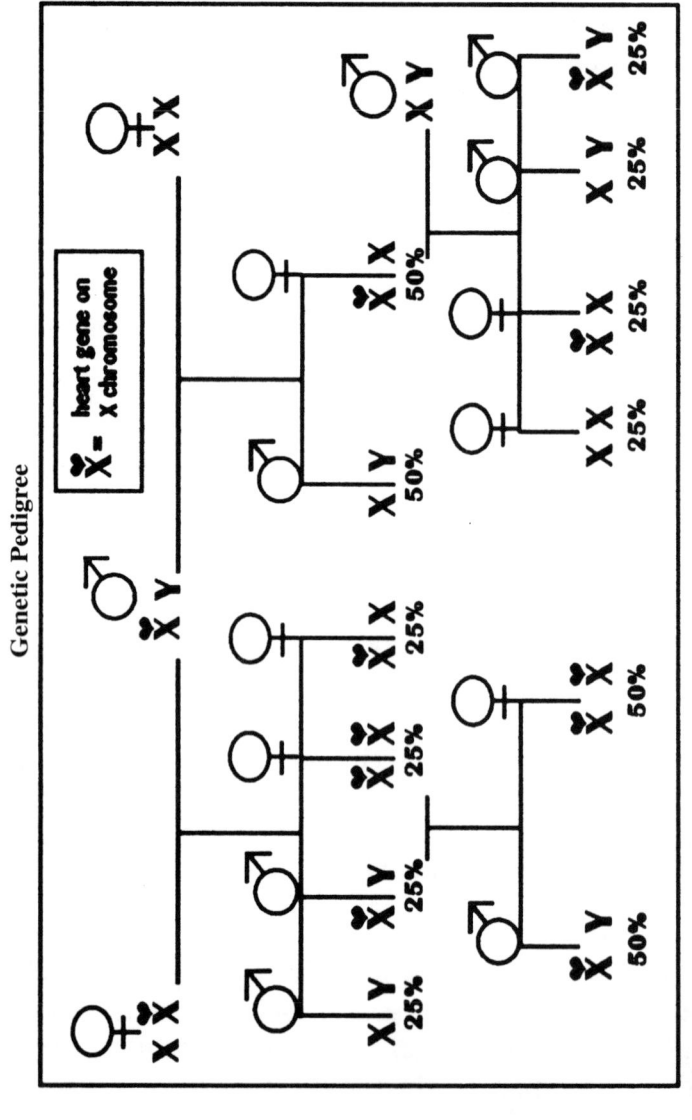

The genetic heart-line pedigree shows the X-factor inheritance pattern for all possible matings.

In studies conducted by Steel and Stewart in 1977 on the inheritance of heart scores in racehorses, an average inheritability of 0.4 was estimated based on inheritance from sire to progeny. Within this study there was a smaller group of Thoroughbreds, in which the heart score of the offspring and both parents had been determined. The group comprised 16 stallions with an average heart score of 123, 51 mares with an average heart score of 115, and 87 progeny - 42 colts with an average heart score of 118 and 45 fillies with an average heart score of 116.

Numbers of Animals, Means, Standard Deviations and Ranges for Heart Score

Observation	Sires	Dams	Male Progeny	Female Progeny
Standardbreds				
All Progeny				
Number	35		221	218
Heart score mean ± S.D.	121.3 ± 6.2		112.5 ± 7.1	111.8 ± 6.4
Heart score range	110-140		96-130	93-130
Progeny with sires and dams				
Number	31	93	93	106
Heart score mean ± S.D.	121.4 ± 6.5	110.0 ± 5.6	113.3 ± 7.1	113.3 ± 6.1
Heart score range	100-140	93-123	6-130	96-130
Thoroughbreds				
All Progeny				
Number	51		192	121
Heart score mean ± S.D.	121.0 ± 5.9		116.4 ± 6.9	113.7 ± 6.5
Heart score range	110-136		100-136	93-130
Progeny with sires and dams				
Number	16	51	42	45
Heart score mean ± S.D.	122.9 ± 5.5	114.9 ± 7.7	118.3 ± 7.1	115.8 ± 6.5
Heart score range	113-133	93-133	106-136	96-130

(reprinted from the Australian Veterinary Journal, Vol 53, July, 1977)

The regression coefficients (statistical method for seeking predictive relationships) obtained between the heart scores of parents and offspring averaged 19 percent from sire to progeny and 59% from dam to progeny. Thus the total of the parent contribution to the heart scores of their progeny was 78 percent.

Since this total could possibly include non-genetic influences from the mare to her foal, the purely genetic heritability is based on her contribution being equal to the sire, i.e., 0.19 + 0.19 = 0.38. This estimate of 38 percent is remarkably close to Cunningham's previous estimate of 35 percent for the inheritance of track performance.

The regressive coefficient from sire to son was 0.06, or statistically zero. From sire to daughter, it was 0.32. From dam to son, it was 0.78, and from dam to daughter, it was 0.40.

The regression coefficients in the Australian study from sire to daughter could be even higher if it is a recessive gene, since the daughters could have the heart gene and not express it. They would be carriers, with the gene on one X chromosome and not on the other. If the X chromosome without the large heart on it was dominant, then they would not express the characteristic, but would still have a 50-50 chance of passing it on to their sons and daughters.

Under this scenario, a daughter of a large-hearted sire like Secretariat, may or may not express the large heart size, but she would have the ability to pass it on to her progeny on a 50-50 basis. If she were a "double copy" (homozygous or one that had the heart gene on both X chromosomes) she would probably express the heart size and could pass it on to all of her progeny, both male and female.

Dr. Anthony Stewart has used his data in a practical way. "I did this with one filly a while ago," he says. "I bought her as a three-year-old that had one start over 1,000 meters. We liked her pedigree. Her family was good back to the third dam, but there was a gap of two generations when the mares hadn't done much. We didn't know why. I told the fellow we would buy her provided her heart score was good. It was, and we have won a stakes race with her already – a Group 3 race. She has come on well."

Stewart said he is surprised about the way buyers are measuring the hearts of yearlings at the major sales in America before purchasing them.

"The heart grows in a horse until the age of three," he said, "so you are guessing a little with yearlings. If they are big at that age, they are fine. But I think they are a bit daring rushing an ultrasound at that age."

More data was needed in order to go beyond the ability to predict the performance of a yearling from measured heart data to the long-sought ability to breed for future champions along established genetic principles.

If that yearling was the product of carefully considered genetic principles in his or her breeding, then the likelihood of a large heart was increased significantly.

Chapter 10

The X Factor

After Sham's death and the discovery of the Princequillo link between him and Secretariat, an intensive pedigree search project was launched combining what the Australians believed about sex linkage and what was learned from geneticists about the characteristics of a sex-linked trait.

Dr. Gus Cothran, a geneticist at the University of Kentucky's Maxwell Gluck Equine Research Center, said that if what the Australians believed was true about sex linkage, then the characteristic was probably a genetic mutation that would trace to a single source.

A genetic mutation, according to Cothran, would not change for hundreds of years. So it was possible that the gene that gave Eclipse, who was foaled in 1764, his large heart, was the same gene that gave Secretariat, foaled in 1970, his large heart.

This search took several months and hundreds of computer hours before a genetic link was found along the X chromosome trail between the two great stallions, separated by more than 200 years of history, through the mare Pocahontas, foaled in England in 1837.

Pocahontas was a mare of rare vitality who lived to be 33 and produced for 20 years. Although not a particularly successful racehorse, Pocahontas demonstrated her extraordinary vitality by finishing second in a field of nine in a race at Chatham, England, in 1842 at a time when she was five months in foal to Camel.

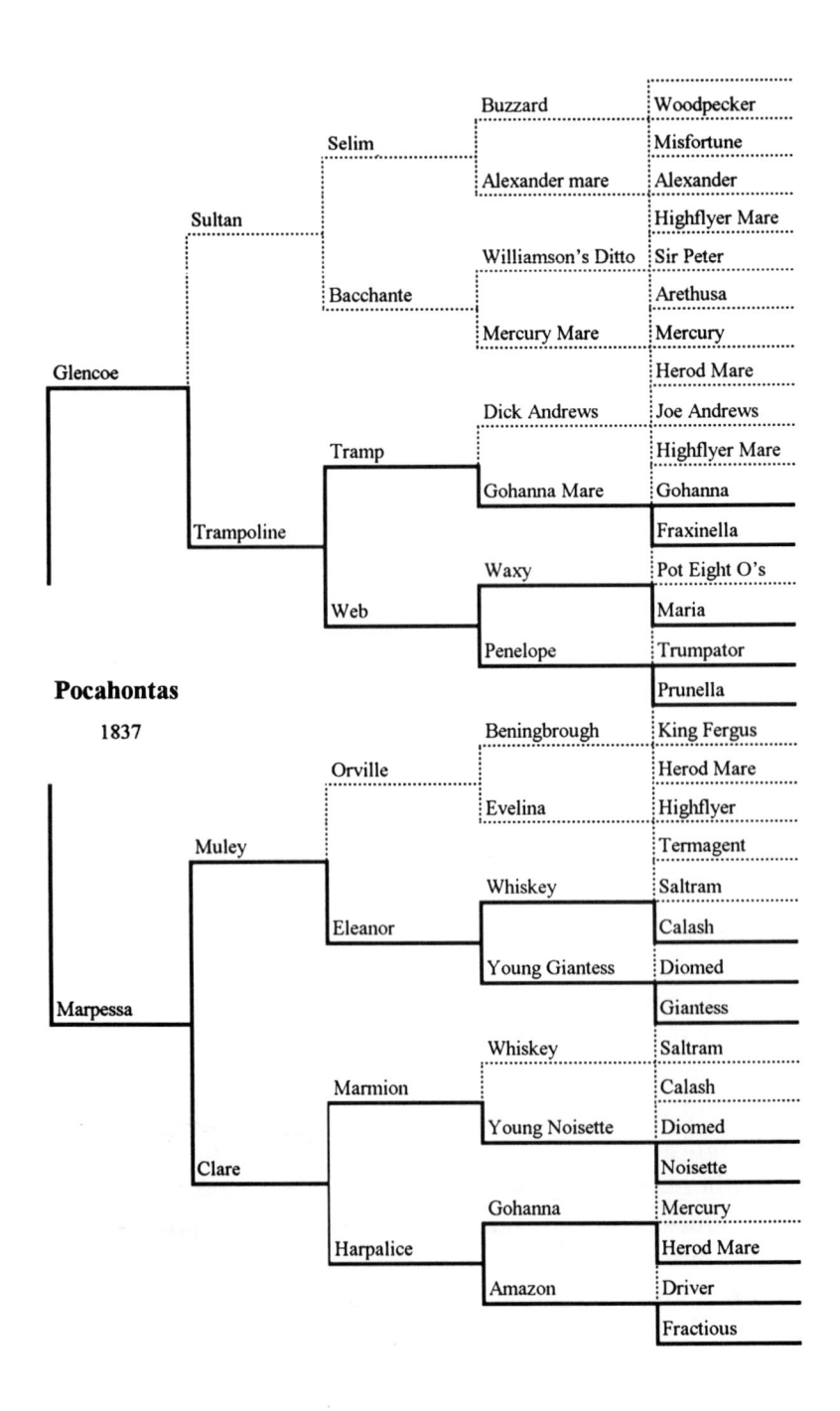

Pocahontas
1837

- Glencoe
  - Sultan
    - Selim
      - Buzzard
        - Woodpecker
        - Misfortune
      - Alexander mare
        - Alexander
        - Highflyer Mare
    - Bacchante
      - Williamson's Ditto
        - Sir Peter
        - Arethusa
      - Mercury Mare
        - Mercury
        - Herod Mare
  - Trampoline
    - Tramp
      - Dick Andrews
        - Joe Andrews
        - Highflyer Mare
      - Gohanna Mare
        - Gohanna
        - Fraxinella
    - Web
      - Waxy
        - Pot Eight O's
        - Maria
      - Penelope
        - Trumpator
        - Prunella

- Marpessa
  - Muley
    - Orville
      - Beningbrough
        - King Fergus
        - Herod Mare
      - Evelina
        - Highflyer
        - Termagent
    - Eleanor
      - Whiskey
        - Saltram
        - Calash
      - Young Giantess
        - Diomed
        - Giantess
  - Clare
    - Marmion
      - Whiskey
        - Saltram
        - Calash
      - Young Noisette
        - Diomed
        - Noisette
    - Harpalice
      - Gohanna
        - Mercury
        - Herod Mare
      - Amazon
        - Driver
        - Fractious

Although she died in 1870 and time makes it impossible to know for sure, from the startling fact that she tracks to Eclipse's daughter, Everlasting, both through her sire, Glencoe, and on her tail-female line through her dam, Marpessa, the chance of her being a double copy mare for the large heart of Eclipse is very probable.

Pocahontas tracks to Everlasting through two daughters of the Woodpecker mare: Fraxinella in Glencoe's pedigree, and Fractious, in Pocahontas' pedigree.

According to geneticist Dr. Gus Cothran, having the same daughter of Eclipse on both the top and bottom of her pedigree probably explains why she has been the main conduit of this characteristic from Eclipse. Given the more than 200 year duration of this genetic trait, it is ironic that it descends from an Eclipse daughter named Everlasting.

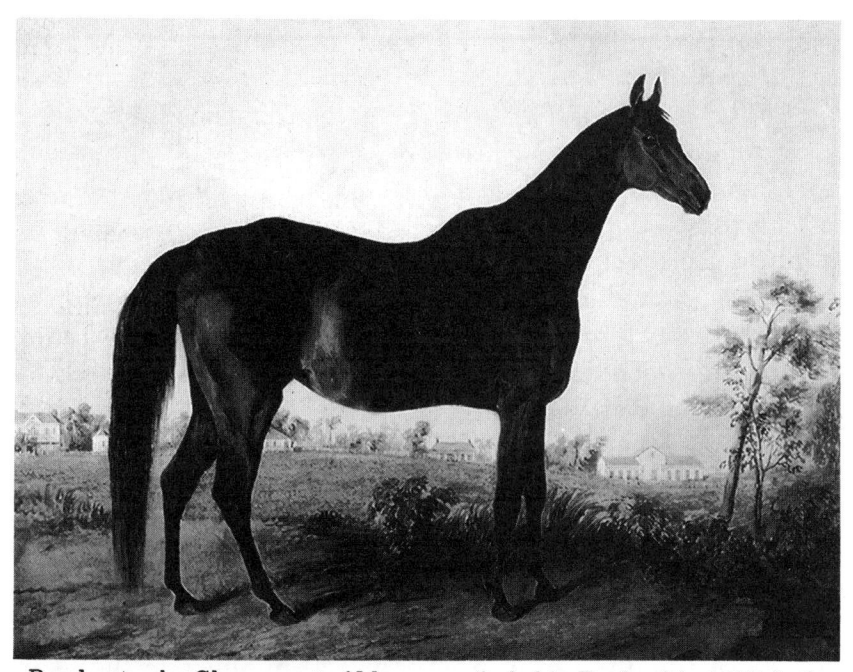

Pocahontas by Glencoe out of Marpessa, foaled in England in 1837, is the genetic link to Eclipse and the large heart.
Painting by Edward Troye courtesy of the Thoroughbred Times

And what progeny she produced! Through her sons, Stockwell, King Tom, Rataplan, and her daughter, Araucaria, Eclipse's great heart found its way down through the centuries. Every large-hearted horse researched traced along the X chromosome trail to this famous ancestress.

The large-hearted horses in Australia, including Phar Lap, follow the X chromosome to Pocahontas and Eclipse. A daughter of Stockwell, Lady Chester was the dam of Chester, a great Australian racehorse and sire. Araucaria produced Apremont, who exercised considerable influence on the bloodstock of New Zealand. Sandal, dam of Instep, ancestress of Aurum, Auraria, Desert Gold, Nadean, and other noted Australian horses, was a daughter of Stockwell.

The genetic link, which was found connecting every large-hearted horse researched through this amazing mare, is called the X-Factor. It is the basis for an ongoing study involving two universities in a search for the genetic marker for the trait.

For more than a year, research has been conducted involving Cothran and Dr. Frederick Fregin, one of the nation's top equine cardiologists and director of the Marion duPont Scott Equine Medical Center at Virginia Tech in Leesburg, Virginia. More than 120 Thoroughbreds, both top and failed racehorses, horses in training and breeding stock, have been measured using electrocardiograms (ECG). Blood samples have been taken from each horse to be used in the DNA research for the genetic marker.

The research goal has been to document a genetic characteristic and establish a pattern of inheritance. Through heart measurements specific large heart lines from sire to daughter to son have been tracked. Specific large heart lines have been measured and consistent heart sizes from the same large-hearted broodmare sires have been found.

According to Cothran, "The initial findings on the heart scores would suggest that the genetic characteristic is probably co-dominant. That means there is a difference between no copy, one copy, and two copies."

After the pattern of inheritance is established on the X chromosome lines, then the formal search for an X-linked marker which affects the heart size is to be launched. Preliminary blood research is already under way. Blood samples taken from each subject are currently being used in the DNA search for a genetic marker.

"If we find what we think we will, and identify the genetic marker, then it will be a matter of a simple blood test to know if an individual has this inheritable characteristic," Cothran said.

In doing the heart measurements for the project, the ECG was used so that the research would be consistent with the heart scores developed in the use of ECGs by Australian researchers. Fregin had met the late Australian, Dr. James D. Steel, who originated the research on large hearts in racehorses, at an international conference in South Africa.

Steel had begun using the electrocardiogram in his research in 1953 and developed the use of the ECGs to determine heart scores. Fregin was very interested in what Steel had discovered using the ECG to measure hearts and about the relationship he was demonstrating between large hearts and performance in racehorses. Fregin has been using the same method of measuring hearts for the past 20 years.

"It is a non-invasive technique for determining heart size," Fregin said. "Dr. Steel and Dr. Anthony Stewart have shown significant correlation between the heart score and racing performance in their research that indicated that a large heart was at least one factor that could be associated with a successful racehorse.

"I am very encouraged by the initial studies that we have done on the mares and stallions."

Steel, of course, had coined the term "heart score" to communicate his findings which he correlated with heart weight, stroke volume, cardiac output, and aerobic power. Hearts are considered large in male horses with heart scores of 120 or more, and in fillies and mares with heart scores of 116 or more. Horses with heart scores of 103 or less are considered small. Those horses with heart scores between the two groups of 104-115 are considered medium or normal-sized hearts.

Since Steel first reported his findings, the relationship between heart scores and performance has been confirmed in both Thoroughbred and Standardbreds by several other groups abroad.

"During galloping, the horse with the large heart may attain cardiac output of at least 200 liters (44 gallons) of blood per minute and the horse with the small heart only about half this volume," said Stewart, one of the leading researchers in the field of heart research from the School of Veterinary Science at the University of Melbourne "The high cardiac output during exercise represents an enormous advantage to the racehorse with the large heart."

The presence of a large heart in a racehorse is not a guarantee of a winner. It is only a piece of the puzzle. There are too many variables in racing for one characteristic to be the "smoking gun" for a champion. But studies show that horses with lower heart scores do not perform as well or as consistently in high class racing as do horses with high heart scores.

Although a large heart is considered an asset in a racehorse, there will always be some horses endowed with other attributes so superb that they may compensate for a disadvantage arising from a slightly smaller heart. Such is the case of superior runners like Bold Ruler and Caro. They made their mark on racing without the advantage of a large heart. And when bred to mares with large hearts, they sired such sons as Secretariat and With Approval.

Heart size will not help a racehorse be a champion if he is unsound, has bad conformation, is not interested in running, is poorly trained, or any number of factors that can impact on the success or failure of a racehorse.

Thoroughbreds have been bred for hundreds of years based on their performance. Because that performance was influenced by the size of their hearts, breeders have been inadvertently breeding for large hearts for centuries, allowing the genetic link to make its way down countless generations. Now, with the genetic knowledge gained in this characteristic, that performance pattern trait can be more selectively bred into the breed.

In the pedigree research for the X-Factor, all large-hearted stallions and mares were found to trace back along the X chromosome trail to Eclipse through the mare Pocahontas. It is probable that the genetic mutation goes even further back somewhere into the desert. But the purpose of this study was to make the connection along a path where there was physical evidence of large hearts.

When Eclipse died, for instance, he had been found to have an extraordinarily large heart. This was the sort of evidence needed.

Using the X-Factor heart line, it has been possible to identify horses which would have large hearts based on their pedigree and horses who would not. The large heart can be followed from sire to daughter to son and to daughter. Full brothers and sisters, third-generations, stallions, broodmares, and horses in training have been measured, and the tests bore out what their pedigrees indicated.

In addition to specific heartlines which seem to also indicate a pattern of performance, the other characteristic besides a large heart found along the X-Factor is that all of the large-hearted sires turned out to be outstanding broodmare sires.

This is understandable because the characteristic passes on the X chromosome so the sire passes it on through his daughters and the dam gives it to her sons and daughters.

This explains why a stallion like Bold Ruler, who had a normal-sized heart, was so successful when coupled with a Princequillo mare carrying the large heart. It also explains that old story of the birth of Secretariat.

When Ogden Phipps, owner of Bold Ruler, and Penny Cheneryflipped a coin to see who would have the first foal in a mating between Bold Ruler and Chenery's mare, Somethingroyal, Phipps won the toss and the first foal – a filly

Mill Reef
1968

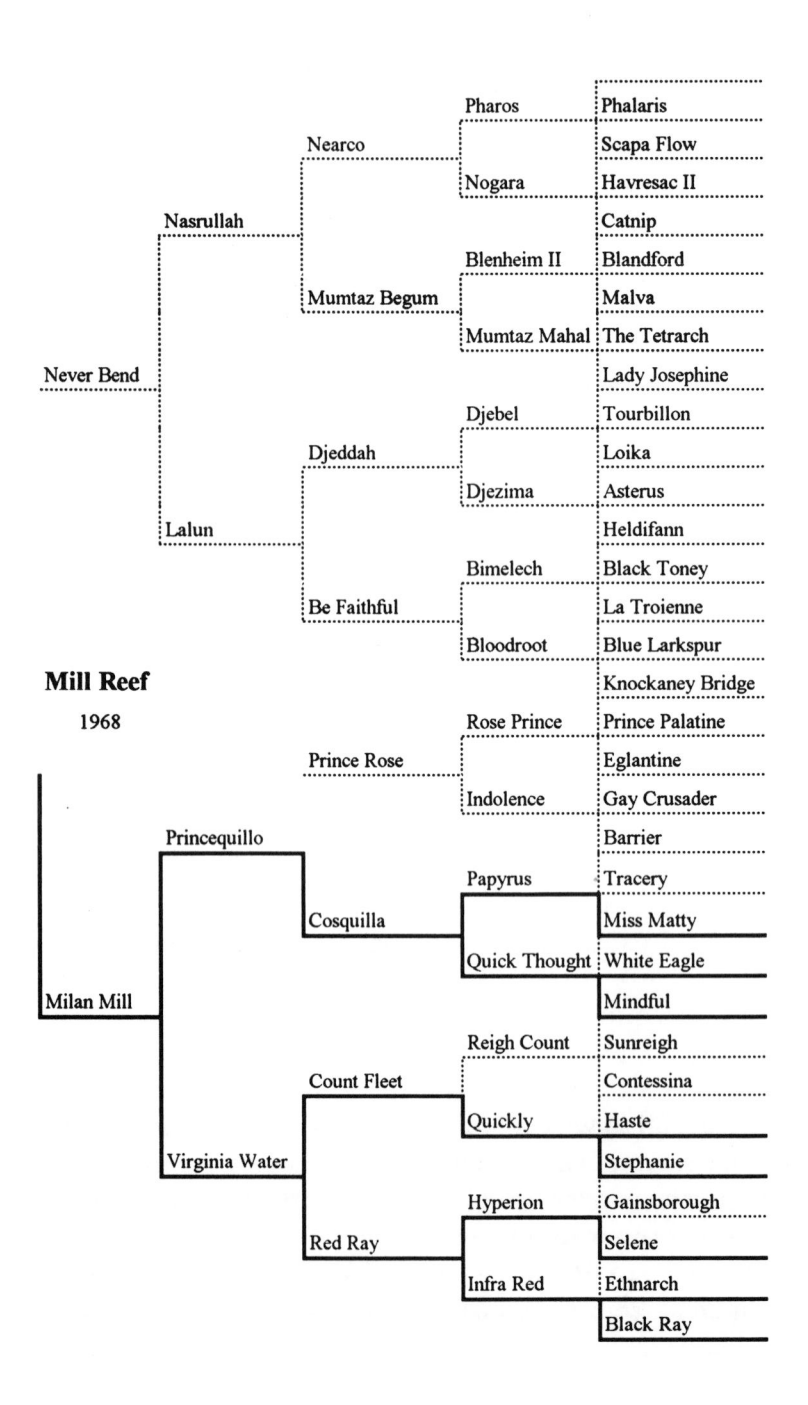

- Never Bend
  - Nasrullah
    - Nearco
      - Pharos
        - Phalaris
        - Scapa Flow
      - Nogara
        - Havresac II
        - Catnip
    - Mumtaz Begum
      - Blenheim II
        - Blandford
        - Malva
      - Mumtaz Mahal
        - The Tetrarch
        - Lady Josephine
  - Lalun
    - Djeddah
      - Djebel
        - Tourbillon
        - Loika
      - Djezima
        - Asterus
        - Heldifann
    - Be Faithful
      - Bimelech
        - Black Toney
        - La Troienne
      - Bloodroot
        - Blue Larkspur
        - Knockaney Bridge

- Milan Mill
  - Princequillo
    - Prince Rose
      - Rose Prince
        - Prince Palatine
        - Eglantine
      - Indolence
        - Gay Crusader
        - Barrier
    - Cosquilla
      - Papyrus
        - Tracery
        - Miss Matty
      - Quick Thought
        - White Eagle
        - Mindful
  - Virginia Water
    - Count Fleet
      - Reigh Count
        - Sunreigh
        - Contessina
      - Quickly
        - Haste
        - Stephanie
    - Red Ray
      - Hyperion
        - Gainsborough
        - Selene
      - Infra Red
        - Ethnarch
        - Black Ray

who inherited her father's heart. The second foal was a colt who inherited his mother's heart and the rest is history.

In the matter of performance, while the large heart is only one piece of the puzzle that makes up a champion racehorse, there are many examples of the characteristic in the most outstanding individuals of the breed.

According to Stewart, "Champion racehorses through the ages have been found to have large hearts, high heart scores, or both. Eclipse, the greatest Thoroughbred of the 18th century, was said to have a heart of 14 pounds, whereas that of the average racehorse today weighs about 8 1/2 pounds."

With the hindsight of autopsy reports, heart size might explain the 1971 mile and a quarter Eclipse Stakes held in July at Sandown Park in England. In that race, another famous Princequillo grandson, Mill Reef, whose autopsy found him to have a 17-pound heart, soundly beat the French champion Caro, who had a normal-sized heart, by four lengths and in course-record time.

In the race, the 3-year-old Mill Reef also faced England's leading older miler, Welsh Pageant, who was trying the distance for the first time. At the start of the race, Welsh Pageant broke on top so quickly that it took a couple of furlongs before either of the expected pacemakers could catch up with him for their appointed role. By six furlongs, Bright Beam had gone by and Quebracho had also moved past Welsh Pageant into second place. Mill Reef was behind Welsh Pageant with Caro breathing down his neck. It was Caro's trainer's plan to track Mill Reef and then try to use him up in a speed duel.

But Mill Reef's jockey, Geoff Lewis, was not about to be caught like that and decided to send Mill Reef on earlier than had been anticipated. To hit the front more than two furlongs out, with Sandown's grinding uphill climb ahead of him was a daunting task, but it was the right answer to the Caro challenge. Caro had nothing left to answer Mill Reef's inexorable stride as the little American-bred galloped away from the field to put him four lengths ahead of Caro and another two and a half lengths further back to Welsh Pageant. With the knowledge that Mill Reef had a heart literally twice the size of Caro, it is easier to understand his ability to climb that hill to victory.

It is ironic that the battle between two heart sizes should occur in the stakes named for the earliest known large-hearted champion, Eclipse.

Mill Reef, who was out of the Princequillo daughter, Milan Mill, had a great three-year-old year. He became only the second horse in history to add the Eclipse Stakes and the King George VI & Queen Elizabeth Stakes to his victory in the 192nd English Derby. It was an accomplishment that Tulyar had performed in the second year of the running of the King George VI & Queen Elizabeth Stakes at Ascot.

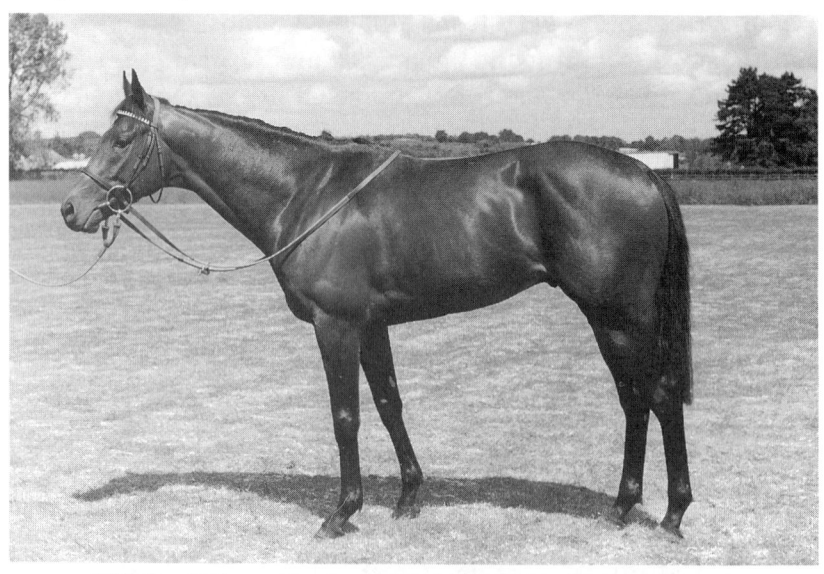

Mill Reef (Never Bend x Milan Mill) had a 17-pound heart
Photo courtesy of the Keeneland Library

During his racing career, Mill Reef was frequently compared to another large-hearted stallion, Nijinsky II. Both stallions, while now dead, are still having their hearts pass down through their daughters, with prominent placings in the top broodmare sire lists.

Chapter 11

Champions and the X-Factor

Such champions as Secretariat, Seattle Slew, Holy Bull, Nijinsky II, Nureyev, Mill Reef, Key to the Mint, Buckpasser, Dr. Fager, Damascus, Northern Dancer, Forty Niner, Spectacular Bid, Woodman, Devil's Bag, Ferdinand, Easy Goer, El Gran Senor, Arrazi, Affirmed, Alysheba, A.P. Indy, Dehere, Whirlaway, Citation, Busher, Tom Fool, War Admiral, Count Fleet, Fort Marcy, Alleged, Crafty Admiral, Swaps, Challedon, Nashua, Native Dancer, Omaha, Silent Screen, Vaguely Noble, Lady's Secret, Gallorette, Crimson Satan, Myrtle Charm, Quill, My Dear Girl, Misty Morn, Mahmoud, Man O' War, Menow, Mocassin, But Why Not, Tom Rolfe, Kelso, With Approval, Unbridled, Sky Classic, Pleasant Colony, Cozzene, Capote, Chief's Crown, Black Tie Affair, Sadler's Wells, and John Henry, to name just a few, all share the characteristic of a large heart.

It is also a characteristic in other successful racehorses who later proved to be a success at stud, such as Princequillo, Blue Larkspur, Storm Cat, Private Account, Seeking the Gold, Danzig, Key to the Kingdom, Halo, Sir Gallahad III, Alydar, Miswaki, Kris S, Polish Navy, Night Shift, Cure the Blues, Fappiano, Storm Bird, Gone West, Rahy, Ogygian, Chief's Crown, Busanda, Believe It, and Myrtlewood, to name just a few.

All of these horses track on the X chromosome line to Eclipse, through the mare Pocahontas. This is what is believed to be the X-Factor Heart Line. In certain lines there are large

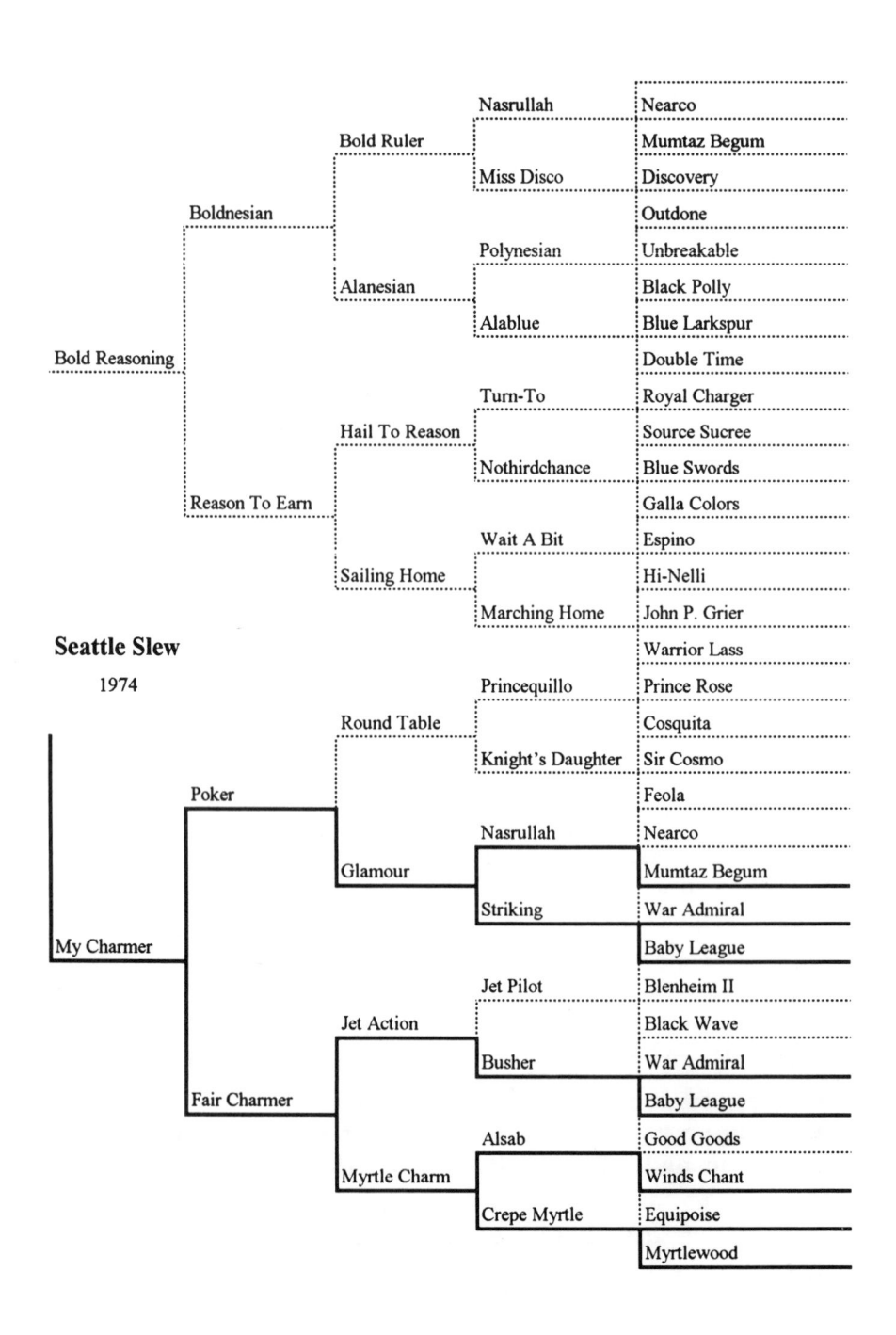

Seattle Slew
1974

- Bold Reasoning
  - Boldnesian
    - Bold Ruler
      - Nasrullah
        - Nearco
        - Mumtaz Begum
      - Miss Disco
        - Discovery
        - Outdone
    - Alanesian
      - Polynesian
        - Unbreakable
        - Black Polly
      - Alablue
        - Blue Larkspur
        - Double Time
  - Reason To Earn
    - Hail To Reason
      - Turn-To
        - Royal Charger
        - Source Sucree
      - Nothirdchance
        - Blue Swords
        - Galla Colors
    - Sailing Home
      - Wait A Bit
        - Espino
        - Hi-Nelli
      - Marching Home
        - John P. Grier
        - Warrior Lass

- My Charmer
  - Poker
    - Round Table
      - Princequillo
        - Prince Rose
        - Cosquita
      - Knight's Daughter
        - Sir Cosmo
        - Feola
    - Glamour
      - Nasrullah
        - Nearco
        - Mumtaz Begum
      - Striking
        - War Admiral
        - Baby League
  - Fair Charmer
    - Jet Action
      - Jet Pilot
        - Blenheim II
        - Black Wave
      - Busher
        - War Admiral
        - Baby League
    - Myrtle Charm
      - Alsab
        - Good Goods
        - Winds Chant
      - Crepe Myrtle
        - Equipoise
        - Myrtlewood

76

hearts. And the one consistent characteristic is the trail back to Pocahontas on the X-lines in their pedigrees.

One of the most notable characteristic in the bloodstock with large hearts is the value of their daughters, when it is found in a sire, and the value of both daughters and sons when it is in the dam. This is because it is a sex-linked characteristic traveling on the X chromosome.

The pattern of performance is seen when this characteristic is passed along the X chromosome starting with a sire such as Secretariat to a daughter like Weekend Surprise to sons like A.P. Indy and Summer Squall.

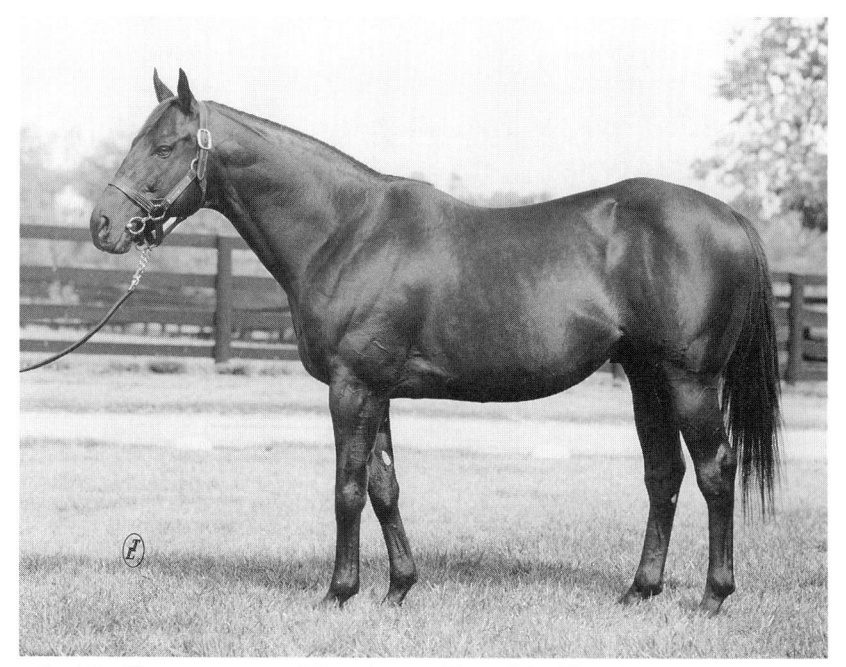

Seattle Slew was named Broodmare Sire of the Year in 1995 and 1996
Photo by Tony Leonard
Courtesy of Three Chimneys Farm

It takes time for the broodmare sire effect to realize itself. A successful large-hearted sire like Seattle Slew, who has sired a number of outstanding sons from such large-hearted mares as Weekend Surprise, dam of A.P. Indy, will not be

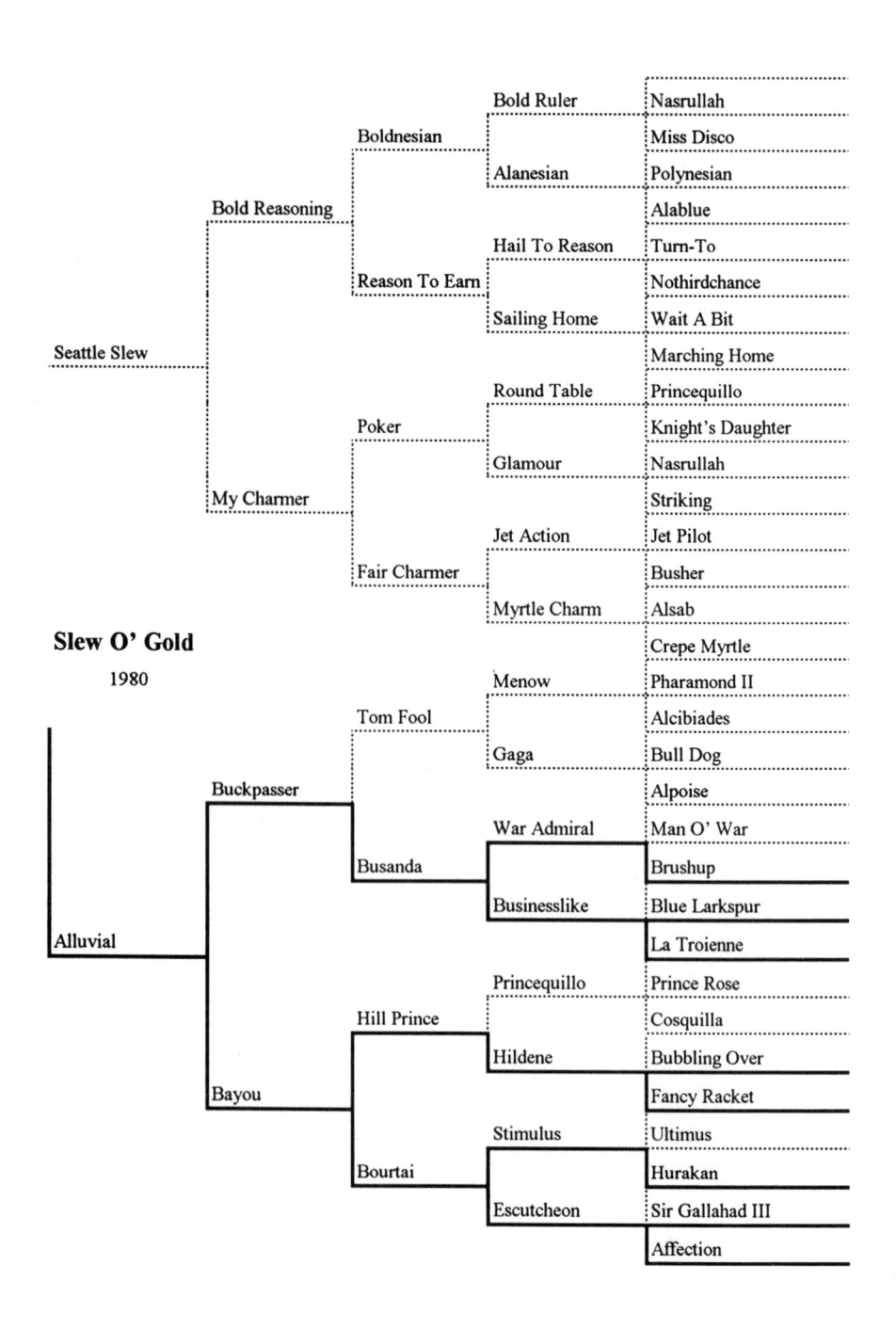

Slew O' Gold
1980

- Seattle Slew
  - Bold Reasoning
    - Boldnesian
      - Bold Ruler
        - Nasrullah
        - Miss Disco
      - Alanesian
        - Polynesian
        - Alablue
    - Reason To Earn
      - Hail To Reason
        - Turn-To
        - Nothirdchance
      - Sailing Home
        - Wait A Bit
        - Marching Home
  - My Charmer
    - Poker
      - Round Table
        - Princequillo
        - Knight's Daughter
      - Glamour
        - Nasrullah
        - Striking
    - Fair Charmer
      - Jet Action
        - Jet Pilot
        - Busher
      - Myrtle Charm
        - Alsab
        - Crepe Myrtle

- Alluvial
  - Buckpasser
    - Tom Fool
      - Menow
        - Pharamond II
        - Alcibiades
      - Gaga
        - Bull Dog
        - Alpoise
    - Busanda
      - War Admiral
        - Man O' War
        - Brushup
      - Businesslike
        - Blue Larkspur
        - La Troienne
  - Bayou
    - Hill Prince
      - Princequillo
        - Prince Rose
        - Cosquilla
      - Hildene
        - Bubbling Over
        - Fancy Racket
    - Bourtai
      - Stimulus
        - Ultimus
        - Hurakan
      - Escutcheon
        - Sir Gallahad III
        - Affection

recognized for his broodmare sire accomplishments until his daughters have time to race and then produce.

But by 1995, when he was selected broodmare sire of the year because of his maternal grandson, Cigar, out of his daughter, Solar Slew, then the path of his large heart and his pattern of performance became clear.

It is interesting to note that the 1996 Three-Year-Old Eclipse champion, Skip Away, who defeated Cigar in the Jockey Club Gold Cup, is carrying the Princequillo heart line through his broodmare sire, Diplomat Way, a maternal grandson of Princequillo. The Princequillo heart is the only heart larger than the War Admiral, which is what Cigar carries courtesy of Seattle Slew.

The best way for a large-hearted sire to pass on his total abilities to a son is to be bred to a large-hearted mare.

Such a mating produced his son, champion Slew O' Gold, who won more than $3.5 million and has sired such large-hearted daughters as: Golden Opinion, the champion 3-year-old filly in France and England and winner of the Coronation Stakes (Eng-1); Gorgeous, winner of $1,171,370 and the Hollywood and Ashland Stakes (Gr-1) and Vanity Invitational Handicap (Gr-1); Tactile, winner of $380,768 and the Gazelle Handicap (Gr-1) and Beldame Stakes (G1); and Sexy Slew, winner of $216,463

To produce Slew O' Gold, Seattle Slew was mated with Alluvial, a daughter of Buckpasser, an outstanding large-hearted sire who carried the large-heart genes of War Admiral through his outstanding daughter, Busanda, who also carried the large heart gene of Blue Larkspur. This mating inbred to the large heart of War Admiral, both top and bottom.

On Seattle Slew's bottom line, his dam, My Charmer, carried War Admiral on the X chromosome line, both through her sire, Poker, who was a maternal grandson to War Admiral's daughter, Striking, and through her dam, Fair Charmer, who was a granddaughter of that great War Admiral daughter, Busher, through her sire, Jet Action.

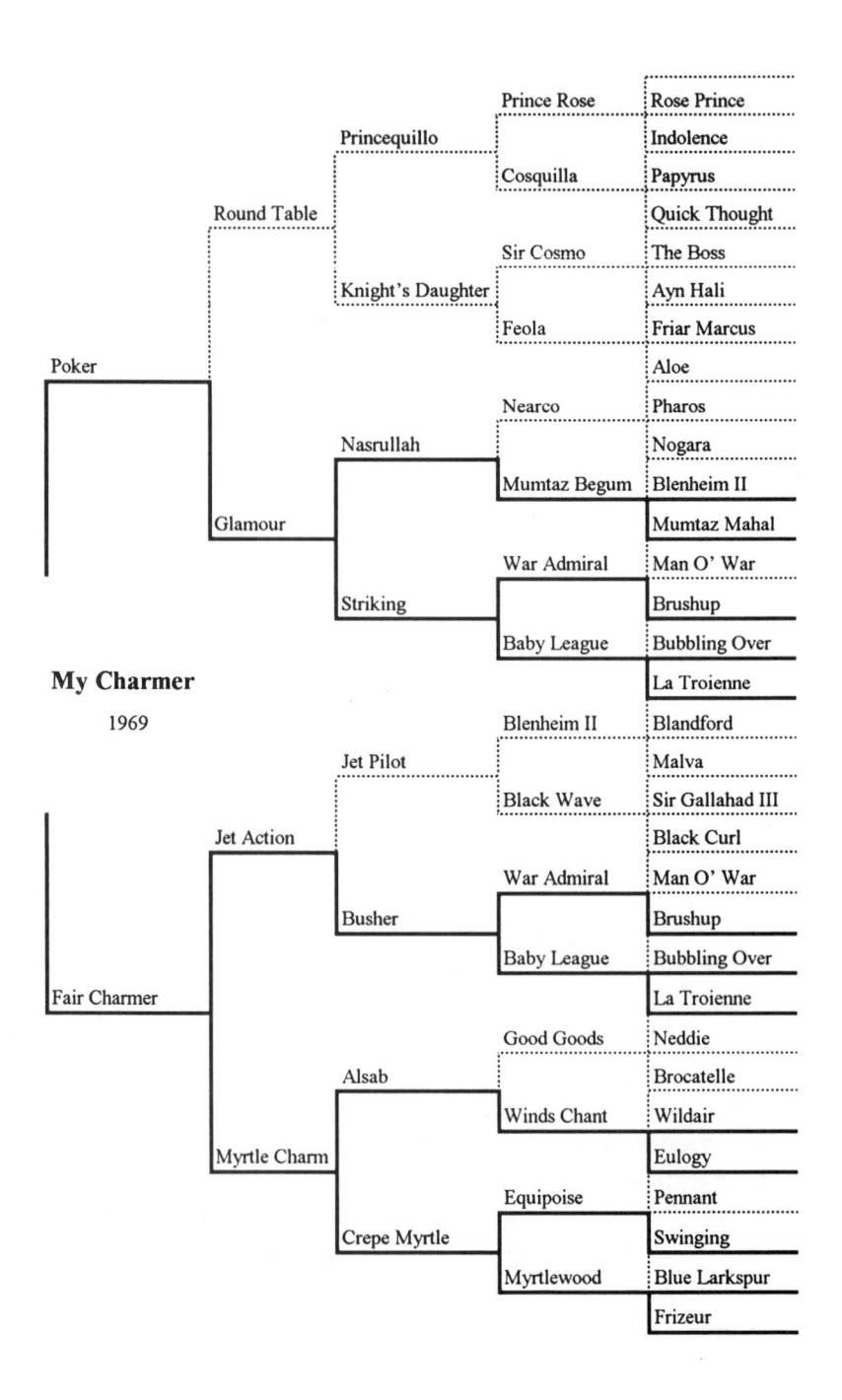

My Charmer
1969

Poker
- Round Table
  - Princequillo
    - Prince Rose
      - Rose Prince
      - Indolence
    - Cosquilla
      - Papyrus
      - Quick Thought
  - Knight's Daughter
    - Sir Cosmo
      - The Boss
      - Ayn Hali
    - Feola
      - Friar Marcus
      - Aloe
- Glamour
  - Nasrullah
    - Nearco
      - Pharos
      - Nogara
    - Mumtaz Begum
      - Blenheim II
      - Mumtaz Mahal
  - Striking
    - War Admiral
      - Man O' War
      - Brushup
    - Baby League
      - Bubbling Over
      - La Troienne

Fair Charmer
- Jet Action
  - Jet Pilot
    - Blenheim II
      - Blandford
      - Malva
    - Black Wave
      - Sir Gallahad III
      - Black Curl
  - Busher
    - War Admiral
      - Man O' War
      - Brushup
    - Baby League
      - Bubbling Over
      - La Troienne
- Myrtle Charm
  - Alsab
    - Good Goods
      - Neddie
      - Brocatelle
    - Winds Chant
      - Wildair
      - Eulogy
  - Crepe Myrtle
    - Equipoise
      - Pennant
      - Swinging
    - Myrtlewood
      - Blue Larkspur
      - Frizeur

But Seattle Slew's large heart must be carried by his daughters. The loss of his champion daughter, Landaluce, was great because of the heart and pattern of performance she might have passed on. But with such Seattle Slew daughters out there as Solar Slew, dam of Cigar; and Grade 1 winners such as Life at the Top, winner of $989,504; Adored, winner of $897,977; Lakeway, winner of $697,020; Seattle Meteor, winner of $397,053; and Le Slew, winner of $402,838, to name just a few, his heart should race on for generations.

Other sires carrying the same heart as Seattle Slew include Seattle Dancer, a son of Nijinsky II out of My Charmer, dam of Seattle Slew. Seattle Dancer, who stands in Japan, has produced such daughters as Via Borghese, winner of $354,797. Another My Charmer son, who currently stands at stud in Italy, is Lomond, by Northern Dancer. Lomond won the Two Thousand Guineas (Eng-1) and his daughters include the Irish champion fillies, Dark Lomond, winner of the Jefferson Smurfit Memorial Irish St. Legers (Ire-1), and Flutter Away, winner of the Moyglare Stud Stakes (Ire-1). He also sired the English champion two- and three-year-old filly, Marling, winner of the English Goffs Irish One Thousand Guineas Stakes (Eng-1) and the Coronation Stakes (Eng-1), and the Italian champion three-year-old filly, Inchmurrin.

A young sire, Desert Secret, whose first foals are yearlings in 1997, has great potential for passing on My Charmer's heart. Desert Secret, a son of Sadler's Wells, is out of Clandestina, a daughter of Secretariat, who was out of My Charmer. When Desert Secret's heart was measured, he was found to have the large heart score consistent with the War Admiral heart.

In doing the heart score measurements for the project, it was found that certain large heart lines were very consistent in heart score, enabling the research team to know which heart line is passed based on the heart score found.

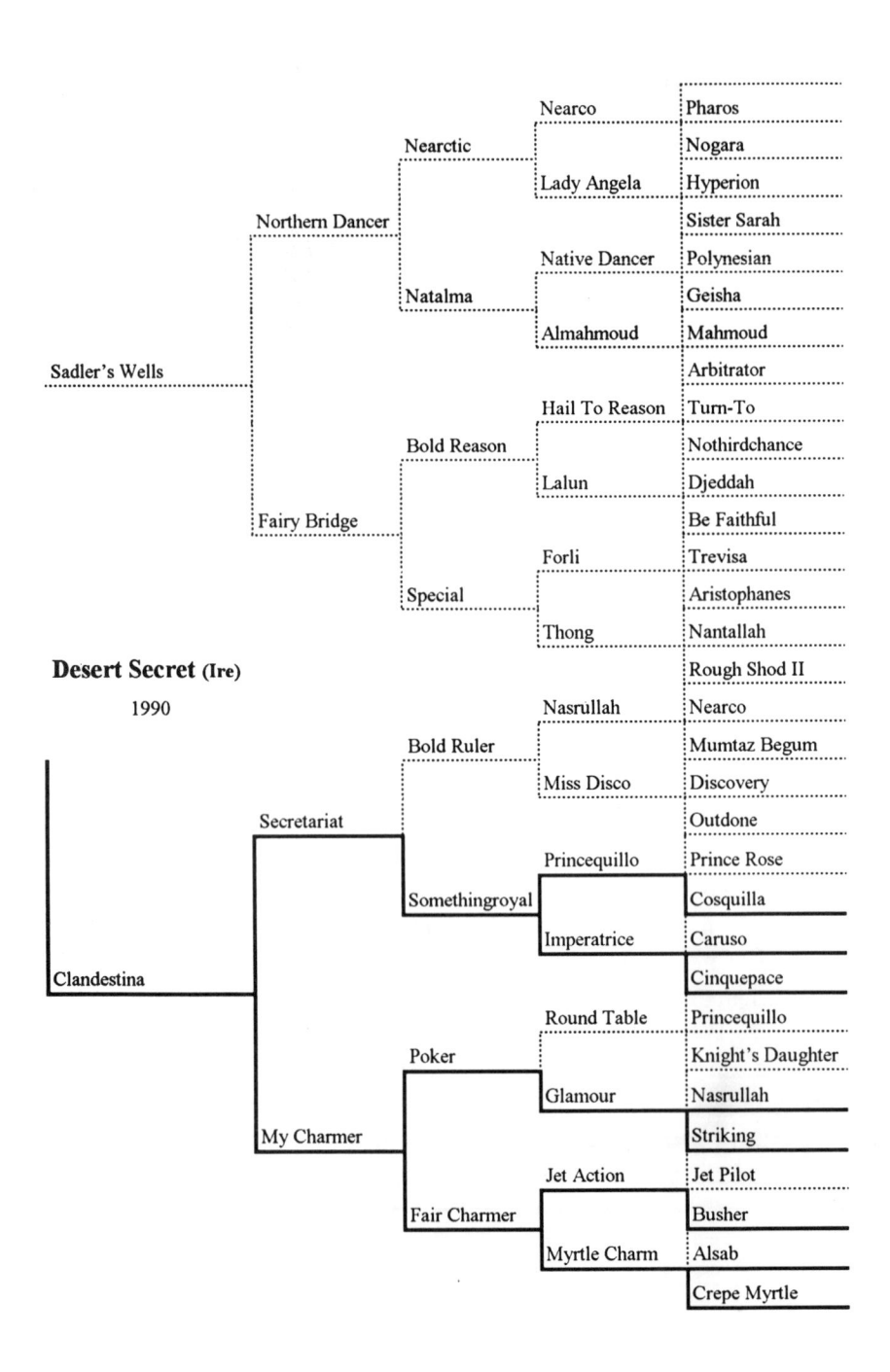

Desert Secret (Ire)
1990

```
                                                  ┌─ Nearco ──────────┬─ Pharos
                                    ┌─ Nearctic ──┤                   └─ Nogara
                                    │             └─ Lady Angela ─────┬─ Hyperion
                  ┌─ Northern Dancer ┤                                └─ Sister Sarah
                  │                 │             ┌─ Native Dancer ───┬─ Polynesian
                  │                 └─ Natalma ───┤                   └─ Geisha
                  │                               └─ Almahmoud ───────┬─ Mahmoud
   ┌─ Sadler's Wells ┤                                                └─ Arbitrator
   │              │                               ┌─ Hail To Reason ──┬─ Turn-To
   │              │                 ┌─ Bold Reason ┤                  └─ Nothirdchance
   │              │                 │             └─ Lalun ───────────┬─ Djeddah
   │              └─ Fairy Bridge ──┤                                 └─ Be Faithful
   │                                │             ┌─ Forli ───────────┬─ Trevisa
   │                                └─ Special ───┤                   └─ Aristophanes
   │                                              └─ Thong ───────────┬─ Nantallah
   │                                                                  └─ Rough Shod II
   │                                              ┌─ Nasrullah ───────┬─ Nearco
   │                                ┌─ Bold Ruler ┤                   └─ Mumtaz Begum
   │                                │             └─ Miss Disco ──────┬─ Discovery
   │              ┌─ Secretariat ───┤                                 └─ Outdone
   │              │                 │             ┌─ Princequillo ────┬─ Prince Rose
   │              │                 └─ Somethingroyal ┤               └─ Cosquilla
   │              │                                  └─ Imperatrice ──┬─ Caruso
   └─ Clandestina ┤                                                   └─ Cinquepace
                  │                                ┌─ Round Table ────┬─ Princequillo
                  │                 ┌─ Poker ──────┤                  └─ Knight's Daughter
                  │                 │              └─ Glamour ────────┬─ Nasrullah
                  └─ My Charmer ────┤                                 └─ Striking
                                    │              ┌─ Jet Action ─────┬─ Jet Pilot
                                    └─ Fair Charmer ┤                 └─ Busher
                                                   └─ Myrtle Charm ───┬─ Alsab
                                                                      └─ Crepe Myrtle
```

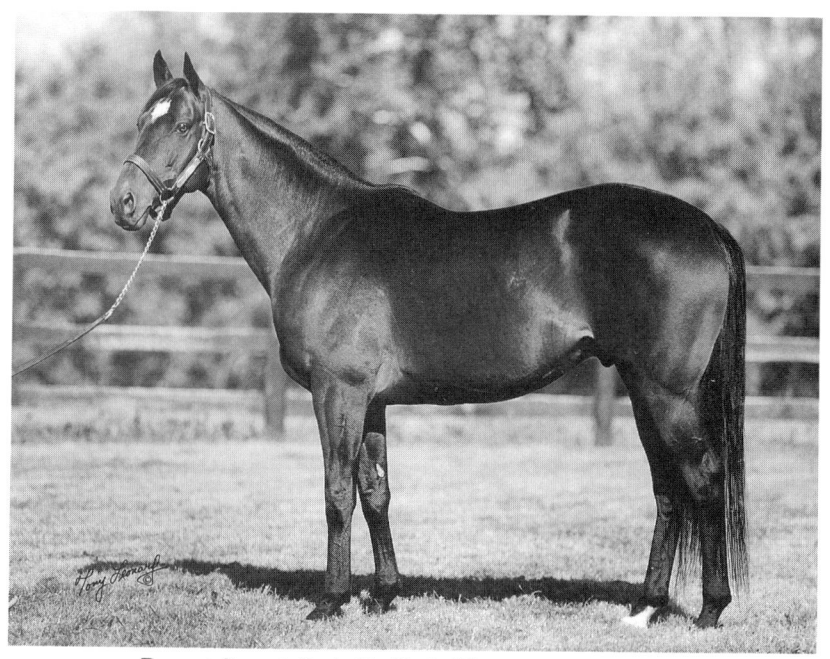

Desert Secret (Ire) (Sadler's Wells x Clandestina)
Photo by Tony Leonard
Courtesy of Crestwood Farm

Sires out of Buckpasser daughters all have large hearts in the same size category. Another large heart line to have similar sized heart scores are sires carrying the Princequillo heart line. The Blue Larkspur heart line, when combined with War Admiral or Princequillo reflects the same size or when standing alone as the heartline. Mahmoud heart lines also seem to measure closely in the large heart category.

Chapter 12

Double Copy Mares

For centuries, breeders have observed the phenomenon of certain sires whose best progeny are females whose produce frequently outperform the preceding generation. These sires are called broodmare sires because they sire dams who produce outstanding individuals.

Genetically speaking, these sires are passing on their best characteristics on the X chromosome, which they can only give their daughters, who in turn can pass on whatever genetic material is on that chromosome to both their sons and daughters.

The large heart found in certain champion racehorses is such a characteristic and may well be one of the prime reasons a sire is considered a broodmare sire. A large-hearted broodmare sire is frequently panned as a sire because he fails to reproduce his brilliance in his sons.

When the characteristic that helped make him a champion is one that only passes on the X chromosome, such as the large heart, this is understandable. Unless the large-hearted sire is mated to a mare with an equally large heart, it is not likely the sire can reproduce his champion status in a son.

Secretariat, who had the world's largest equine heart, was such a sire. His huge engine, which powered him to so many victories, the Triple Crown, Horse of the Year, and track records, could only be inherited by his daughters. Because of this, many declared him a bust as a sire, only later in his life

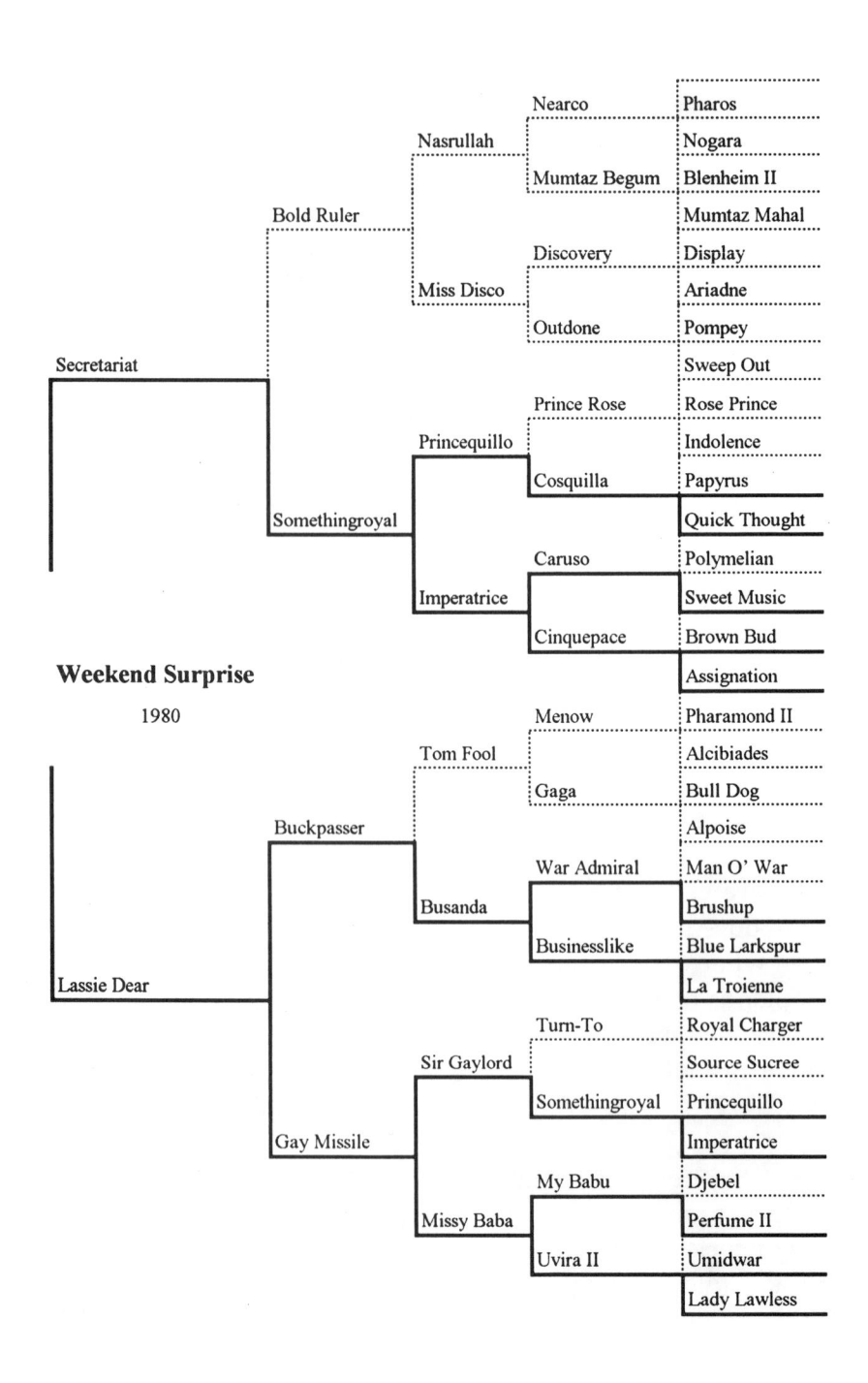

Weekend Surprise
1980

- Secretariat
  - Bold Ruler
    - Nasrullah
      - Nearco
        - Pharos
        - Nogara
      - Mumtaz Begum
        - Blenheim II
        - Mumtaz Mahal
    - Miss Disco
      - Discovery
        - Display
        - Ariadne
      - Outdone
        - Pompey
        - Sweep Out
  - Somethingroyal
    - Princequillo
      - Prince Rose
        - Rose Prince
        - Indolence
      - Cosquilla
        - Papyrus
        - Quick Thought
    - Imperatrice
      - Caruso
        - Polymelian
        - Sweet Music
      - Cinquepace
        - Brown Bud
        - Assignation

- Lassie Dear
  - Buckpasser
    - Tom Fool
      - Menow
        - Pharamond II
        - Alcibiades
      - Gaga
        - Bull Dog
        - Alpoise
    - Busanda
      - War Admiral
        - Man O' War
        - Brushup
      - Businesslike
        - Blue Larkspur
        - La Troienne
  - Gay Missile
    - Sir Gaylord
      - Turn-To
        - Royal Charger
        - Source Sucree
      - Somethingroyal
        - Princequillo
        - Imperatrice
    - Missy Baba
      - My Babu
        - Djebel
        - Perfume II
      - Uvira II
        - Umidwar
        - Lady Lawless

granting him broodmare sire status. Yet, today, his heart is racing via the produce of his daughters, to great racing success.

In passing the large heart on the X chromosome, it is possible for a daughter of a large-hearted sire like Secretariat to be a single copy. That is, a mare who may or may not express the large heart, but who "carries" the large-hearted characteristic on the X chromosome she inherited from her sire. That means she would have a 50-50 chance of passing the large heart gene on to her sons and daughters. In the case of daughters, the dominant X they express could come either from the sire or the dam. With sons, it will always come from the mother.

If a mare is a double copy (a homozygous or one that had the heart gene on both X chromosomes), she would probably express the heart size and pass the gene on to all of her progeny, both male and female. If a characteristic comes on the X chromosome to a son, it is nearly always expressed. But that is not necessarily so in the female. There it depends on which X is dominant.

A modern example of a "double copy" mare is Weekend Surprise. Weekend Surprise is a large-hearted mare who carries the large-heart gene on both of her X chromosomes. She was an outstanding race mare, a graded-stakes winner with earnings of $402,892. Her dam, Lassie Dear, a daughter of the large-hearted sire, Buckpasser, is also a double copy individual.

Weekend Surprise passed on her great heart to sons, champion A.P. Indy, Horse of the Year and winner of more than $2.9 million, and Summer Squall, winner of more than $1.8 million. Those two individuals are now sires passing that heart on to their daughters.

John Henry, who as a gelding was never bred, has been measured and found to have a heart 25% larger than normal. In his pedigree, that many for years have called undistinguished, he has many links to Pocahontas on the bottom side, including those through the very good broodmare sire, Double Jay.

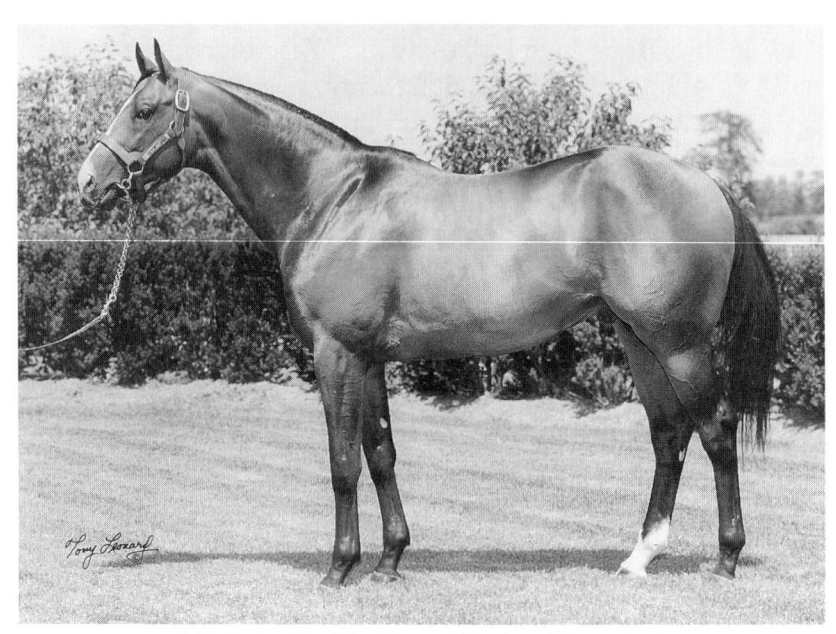

A.P. Indy (Seattle Slew x Weekend Surprise)

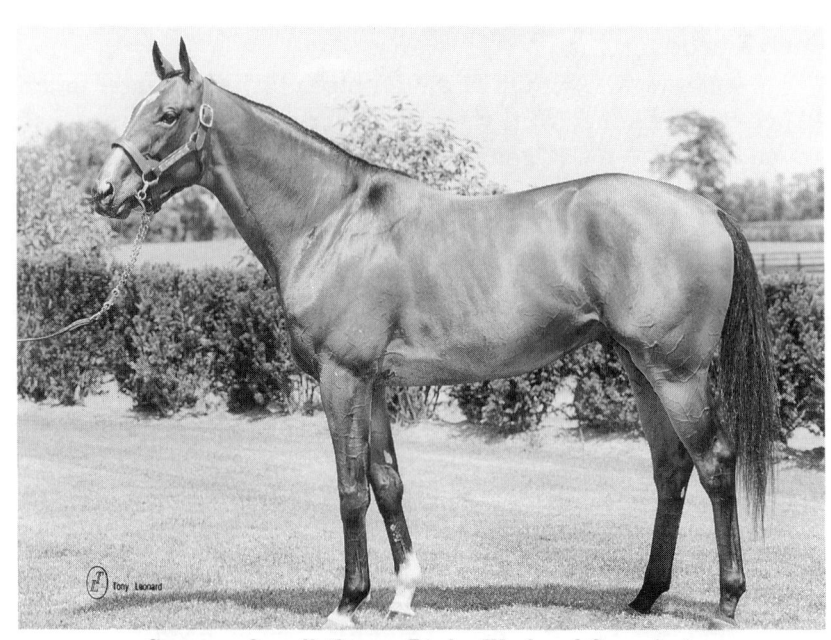

Summer Squall (Storm Bird x Weekend Surprise)

Photos by Tony Leonard
Courtesy of Lane's End Farm

The list of possible double copy mares reads like a "Who's Who" of outstanding broodmares.

Double Copy Mares

Alcibiades	Alluvial	Almahmoud	Althea
Araucaria	Aspidistra	Baby League	Bathing Girl
Be Faithful	Bee Mac	Bel Sheba	Belthazar
Betty's Secret	Bird Flower	Black Helen	Bloodroot
Blue Banner	Blue Denim	Boat	Boudoir II
Bramalea	Broadway	Brushup	Busanda
Busher	Businesslike	Cap and Bells	Chapel of Dreams
Con Game	Cosmah	Cosquilla	Courtly Dee
Crimson Saint	Fall Aspen	Flaming Page	Flitabout
Flower Bowl	Gaga	Gana Facil	Gay Missle
Glorious Song	Hopespringseternal	Imperatrice	Kerala
Key Bridge	Killaloe	La Troienne	Lady Angela
Lady Josephine	Mah Mahal	Maplejinsky	Milan Mill
Millicent	Miss Carmie	Miss Zigby	Misty Morn
Mocassin	Mumtaz Begum	Mumtaz Mahal	My Charmer
My Dear Girl	Myrtlewood	Natalma	Naval Orange
Noble Lassie	Numbered Account	Personal Ensign	Plucky Liege
Prayer Bell	Quickly	Rare Mint	Relaxing
Romanella	Rough Shod II	Secretame	Selene
Sequence	Sharon Brown	Shy Dawn	Six Crowns
Solar Slew	Somethingroyal	South Ocean	Special
Strike a Balance	Striking	Sweet Tooth	Tamerett
Teleran	Terlingua	Toll Booth	Wavy Navy
Won't Tell You			

One of the most important things we have learned is the importance of the dam in producing outstanding racehorses. While following the large heart along the heart lines in the pedigrees of the horses measured, going from sire to dam to daughter and son, it appeared there might be something else happening along the X chromosome.

In many cases there seemed to be a body type that passed from sire to daughter to son. The outstanding broodmare sire, Princequillo, gave certain physical characteristics, besides a large heart, to his daughters. In comparing conformation pictures of Princequillo with daughters Somethingroyal and Key Bridge, there is an

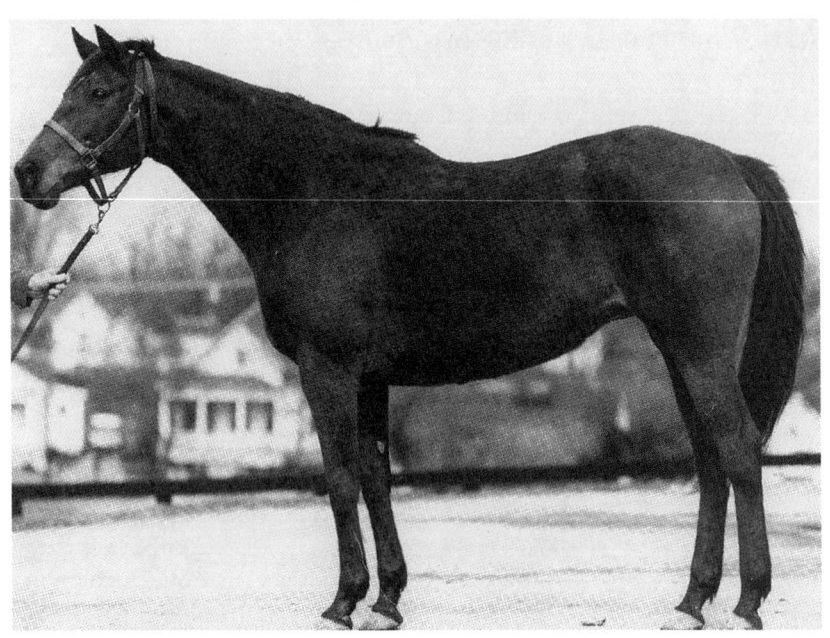

Somethingroyal (Princequillo x Imperatrice)
Photo courtesy of Penny Chenery

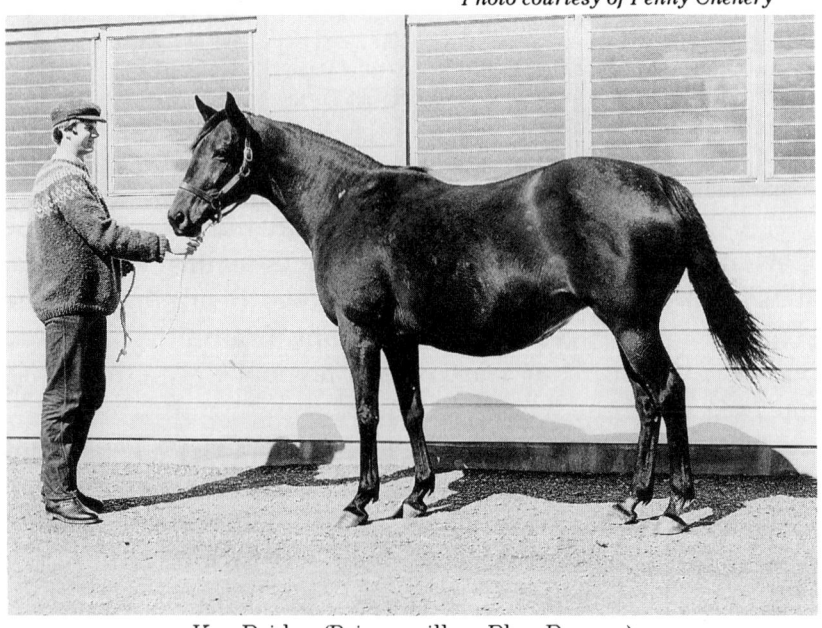

Key Bridge (Princequillo x Blue Banner)
Photo courtesy of Paul Mellon

amazing similarity. Besides the overall conformation likeness, there are certain physical characteristics that show up as well, including unusually small ears and a flat broad face at the top of the skull, that is eerily reflected in daughters of Moscow Ballet and in himself, a maternal grandson of a Princequillo daughter, Milan Mill.

There is an amazing similarity in conformation between Princequillo and daughters Somethingroyal and Key Bridge. Besides overall body type, certain similar physical characteristics including unusually small ears and shape of the head are evident.

They are the same physical characteristics found in Secretariat. When Penny Chenery, owner of Secretariat, first saw the picture of The Last Red, a twin daughter of Moscow Ballet, which is being used in a breeding experiment for the project, because of her very large heart , she said, "Why those are Secretariat's ears!"

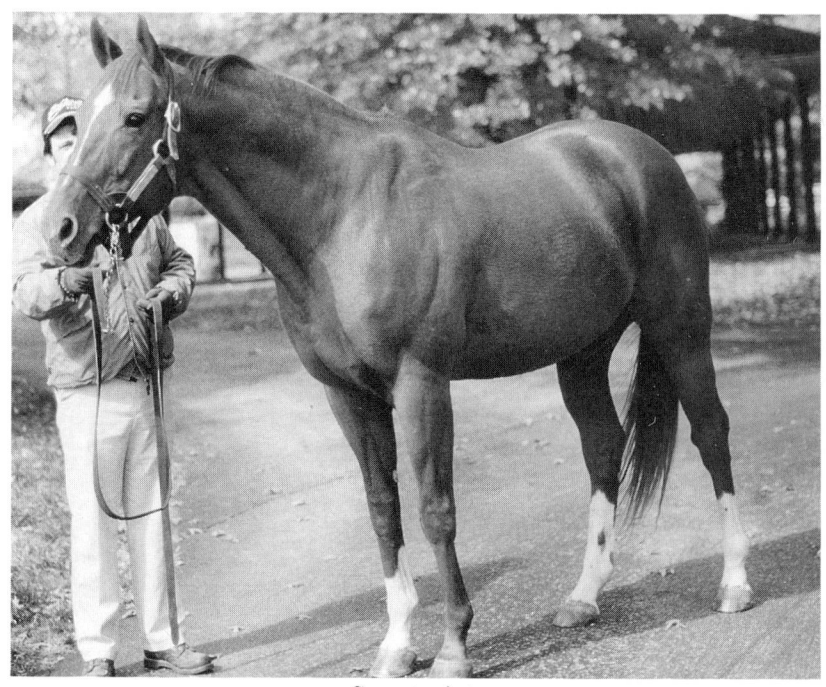

Secretariat

Photo courtesy of Marianna Haun

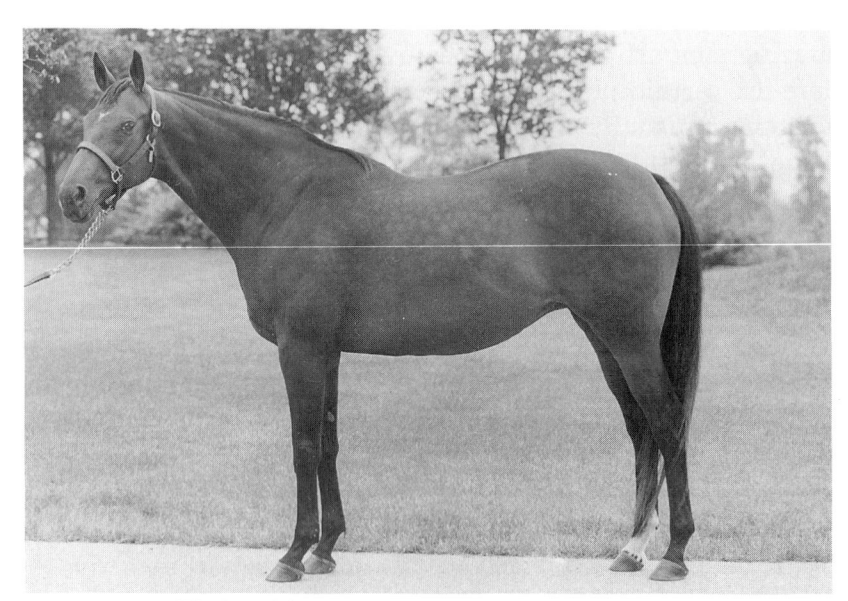

Weekend Surprise (Secretariat x Lassie Dear)
Courtesy of Photos by Z

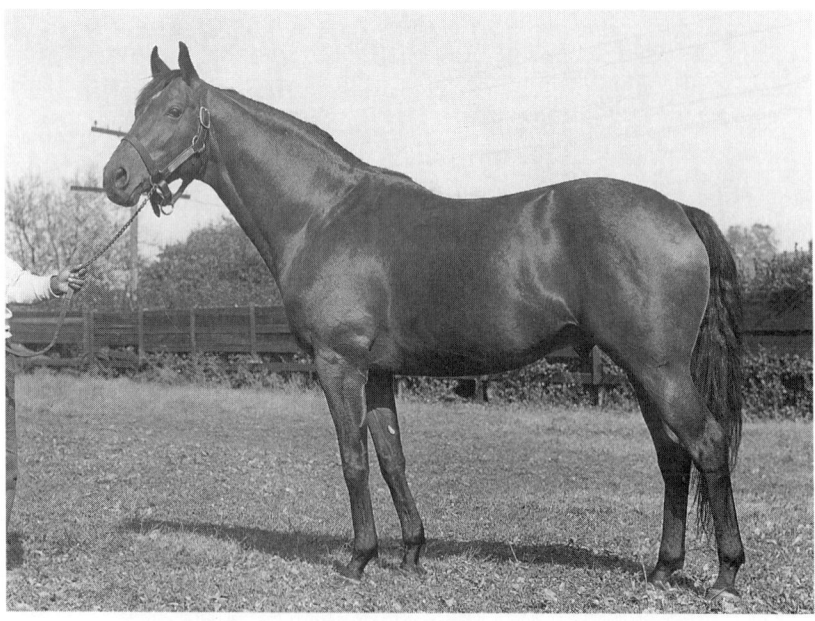

Princequillo (Prince Rose x Cosquilla)
The similarity between Princequillo and Weekend Surprise is striking.
Photo courtesy of the Keeneland Library

Following her recognition of certain physical characteristics in the twin filly, a photographic comparison was made, and those small ears and wide flat forehead, along with sloping shoulders and chest and neck similarities were found to go back to Princequillo, and on to his daughters, and to his maternal grandsons, Secretariat, Moscow Ballet, Mill Reef, and Key to the Mint. When comparing conformation shots of Princequillo and Weekend Surprise, the similarity, especially in the front half of the two horses is very striking.

Genetic studies at Cornell University have now found that in the forming of the horse, the Y chromosome is responsible for the uterine environment and the X chromosome is responsible for the forming of the body of the individual. This is ironic in terms of the male chromosome being in charge of the housekeeping, and the female chromosome being in charge of the formation of the horse inside that environment.

This is an area that needs more research, but it is certainly fascinating. Geneticists have long felt there was something in the sex linkage of physical characteristics passed along the X chromosome. In humans, daughters often more closely resemble their father's family on the maternal side, and sons frequently resemble their mother's side of the family. A classic example is the children of President John F. Kennedy. The daughter, Caroline, resembles her father, and the son, John F. Kennedy Jr., resembles his mother.

A scientific paper released June 28, 1996, from Hunter Genetics in New South Wales, Australia, contends that intelligence is also passed along the X chromosome, in much the same manner as the large heart is passed.

In a paper published in the British medical journal, *The Lancet,* Professor Gillian Turner wrote that there is growing evidence that several key genes for intelligence (and retardation) are found on the X chromosome - the one inherited from the mother.

Turner writes that these genes are distributed along the whole length of the X chromosome and coded for "various anatomical or functional parts of the neural substratum of intelligence."

Under Turner's theory, the smart genes are on the X chromosome, which means a single mutation will have more effect on a man than on a woman because he only gets one X chromosome. Because a woman inherits two X chromosomes, one from her father and one from her mother, any mutation inherited from one may be weakened by the other, unless the smart gene is on both X chromosomes.

This is similar to the circumstances of the large-heart gene. Given the similarity of the genetic structures of all mammals, it also raises some interesting ideas about how temperament and intelligence might be inherited in horses.

Radiologist Norman Rantanen, who developed the ultrasound to measure hearts in the early 1980s, and has since measured more than 3,000 horses, said he has recognized body types along the X chromosome line, although he has not matched up pedigree lines with body types.

"There is a similarity in body type in the large-hearted horses," Rantanen said. "But if they all descend from a single source, there is bound to be a similarity in body type along the X chromosome line," he said.

The principals of heredity were first discovered in 1860 by Mendal, geneticist Gus Cothran said. "That was the beginning of Mendelian genetics. But it wasn't until 1900 that those principals were 'rediscovered' and became a part of our world. So it is really a product of this century. DNA was not recognized as the material of heredity until the 1950s."

In 1919, Dr. Thomas Hunt Morgan of the University of Kentucky, discovered the X and Y chromosome and sex-linked characteristics. He won the Nobel Prize for his discovery.

"He discovered sex linkage using fruit flies," Cothran said. "Based on his work, people began to recognize it in other things, including humans and horses.

"Today more and more research is being conducted on the genetic makeup of both man and horse. We are involved, here at the University of Kentucky in creating a genetic map of the horse. We are basing much of what we know from the research done in the human genome project. Because, genetically speaking, the human mammal and the equine mammal are very similar.

"What we learn about the horse can be of use in human research and what is learned about human genes can have an impact on equine research. What we are finding out about the large heart in some racehorses being a sex-linked characteristic on the X chromosome may be of significant interest to human heart researchers."

The X Factor was identified. What remains is to identify and catalogue the bearers. While all large-hearted horses measured in this project track on the X chromosome trail to Eclipse through the legendary mare Pocahontas, four heart lines seem to produce the largest and most consistent heart scores and which are found in some of the greatest of our modern sires and dams.

The four lines are: Princequillo, arguably this century's greatest broodmare sire; War Admiral, Man O' War's greatest son; Blue Larkspur; and Mahmoud. These four stallions each earned spots on the top broodmare sire lists for more than a decade and their hearts are racing today through the produce of their extraordinary daughters.

PART IV

THE GREAT LINES

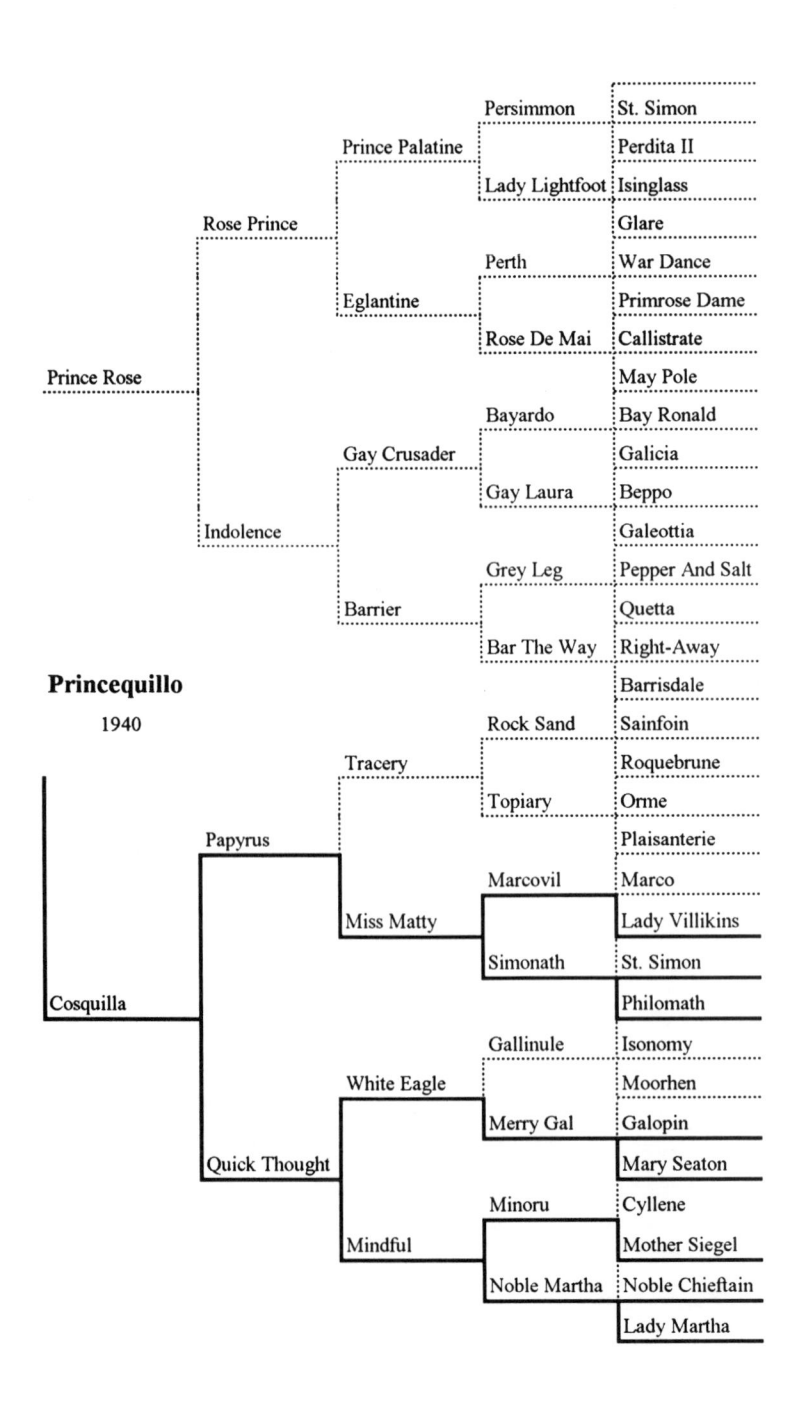

Princequillo
1940

Prince Rose	Rose Prince	Prince Palatine	Persimmon → St. Simon
			Persimmon → Perdita II
			Lady Lightfoot → Isinglass
			Lady Lightfoot → Glare
		Eglantine	Perth → War Dance
			Perth → Primrose Dame
			Rose De Mai → Callistrate
			Rose De Mai → May Pole
	Indolence	Gay Crusader	Bayardo → Bay Ronald
			Bayardo → Galicia
			Gay Laura → Beppo
			Gay Laura → Galeottia
		Barrier	Grey Leg → Pepper And Salt
			Grey Leg → Quetta
			Bar The Way → Right-Away
			Bar The Way → Barrisdale
Cosquilla	Papyrus	Tracery	Rock Sand → Sainfoin
			Rock Sand → Roquebrune
			Topiary → Orme
			Topiary → Plaisanterie
		Miss Matty	Marcovil → Marco
			Marcovil → Lady Villikins
			Simonath → St. Simon
			Simonath → Philomath
	Quick Thought	White Eagle	Gallinule → Isonomy
			Gallinule → Moorhen
			Merry Gal → Galopin
			Merry Gal → Mary Seaton
		Mindful	Minoru → Cyllene
			Minoru → Mother Siegel
			Noble Martha → Noble Chieftain
			Noble Martha → Lady Martha

Chapter 13

Princequillo

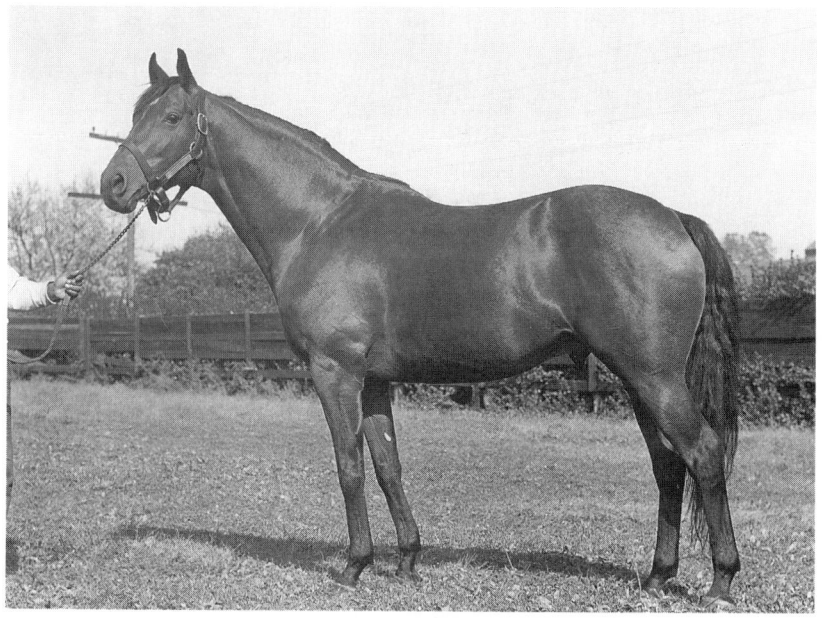

Princequillo, Bay Horse, 1940 (Prince Rose x Cosquilla)
Photo courtesy of the Keeneland Library

The Princequillo Line

In measuring the four lines, the heart scores for Princequillo line stallions were consistently the largest ones found.

In the more than 120 horses measured for the project, the largest heart score found was in the champion Key to the Mint, whose dam, Key Bridge, had the unique pedigree that

Key To The Mint
1969

Graustark	Ribot	Tenerani	Bellini	Cavaliere d'Arpino
				Bella Minna
			Tofanella	Apelle
				Try Try Again
		Romanella	El Greco	Pharos
				Gay Gamp
			Barbara Burrini	Papyrus
				Bucolic
	Flower Bowl	Alibhai	Hyperion	Gainsborough
				Selene
			Teresina	Tracery
				Blue Tit
		Flower Bed	Beau Pere	Son-In-Law
				Cinna
			Boudoir II	Mahmoud
				Kampala
Key Bridge	Princequillo	Prince Rose	Rose Prince	Prince Palatine
				Eglantine
			Indolence	Gay Crusader
				Barrier
		Cosquilla	Papyrus	Tracery
				Miss Matty
			Quick Thought	White Eagle
				Mindful
	Blue Banner	War Admiral	Man O' War	Fair Play
				Mahubah
			Brushup	Sweep
				Annette K.
		Risque Blue	Blue Larkspur	Black Servant
				Blossom Time
			Risque	Stimulus
				Risky

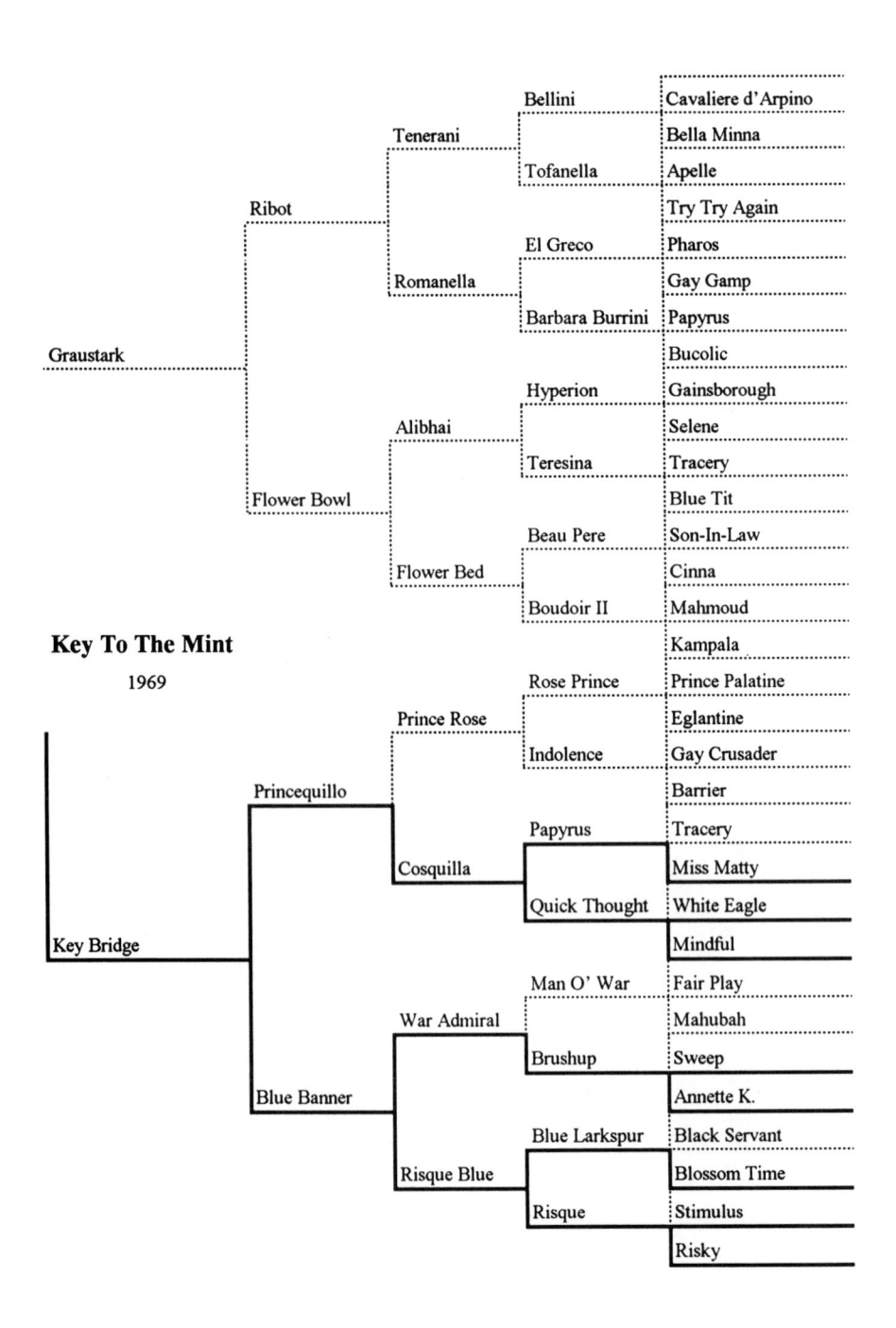

contained three of the largest heart lines: Princequillo, War Admiral, and Blue Larkspur.

Key Bridge, who was unraced, had eight runners from 11 foals, with seven winners and four stakes winners. She was a daughter of Princequillo out of the double copy mare Blue Banner, a stakes winner of $121,175, who had nine runners from 11 foals, with seven winners and one stakes winner.

Blue Banner was a daughter of War Admiral out of the Blue Larkspur daughter, Risque Blue, who was unraced, but produced 10 runners from 14 foals with seven winners and two stakes winners.

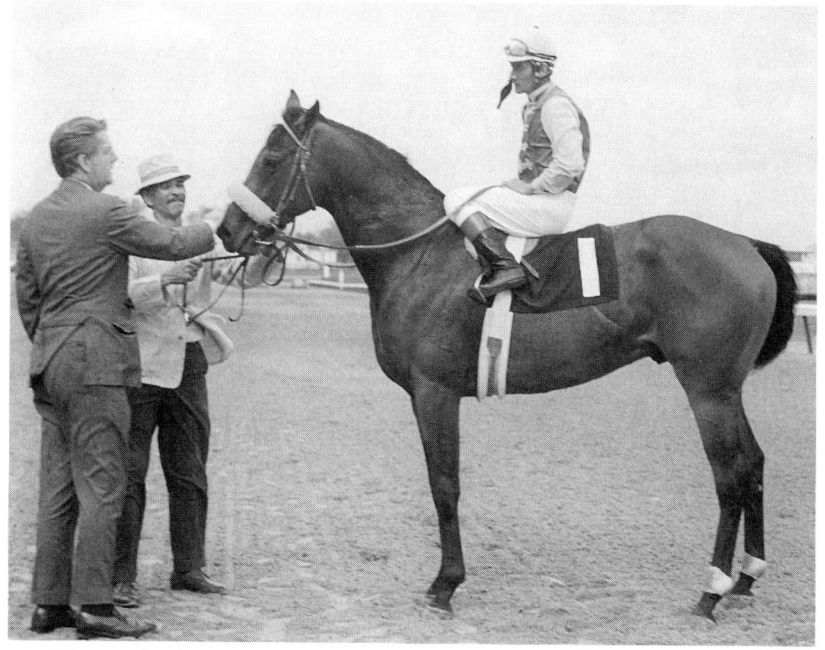

Key to the Mint's pedigree contains the three largest-heart lines
Photo courtesy of Paul Mellon

In addition to Key to the Mint, Key Bridge also produced Horse of the Year, Fort Marcy, who unfortunately was gelded, so we will never know what he might have sired.

101

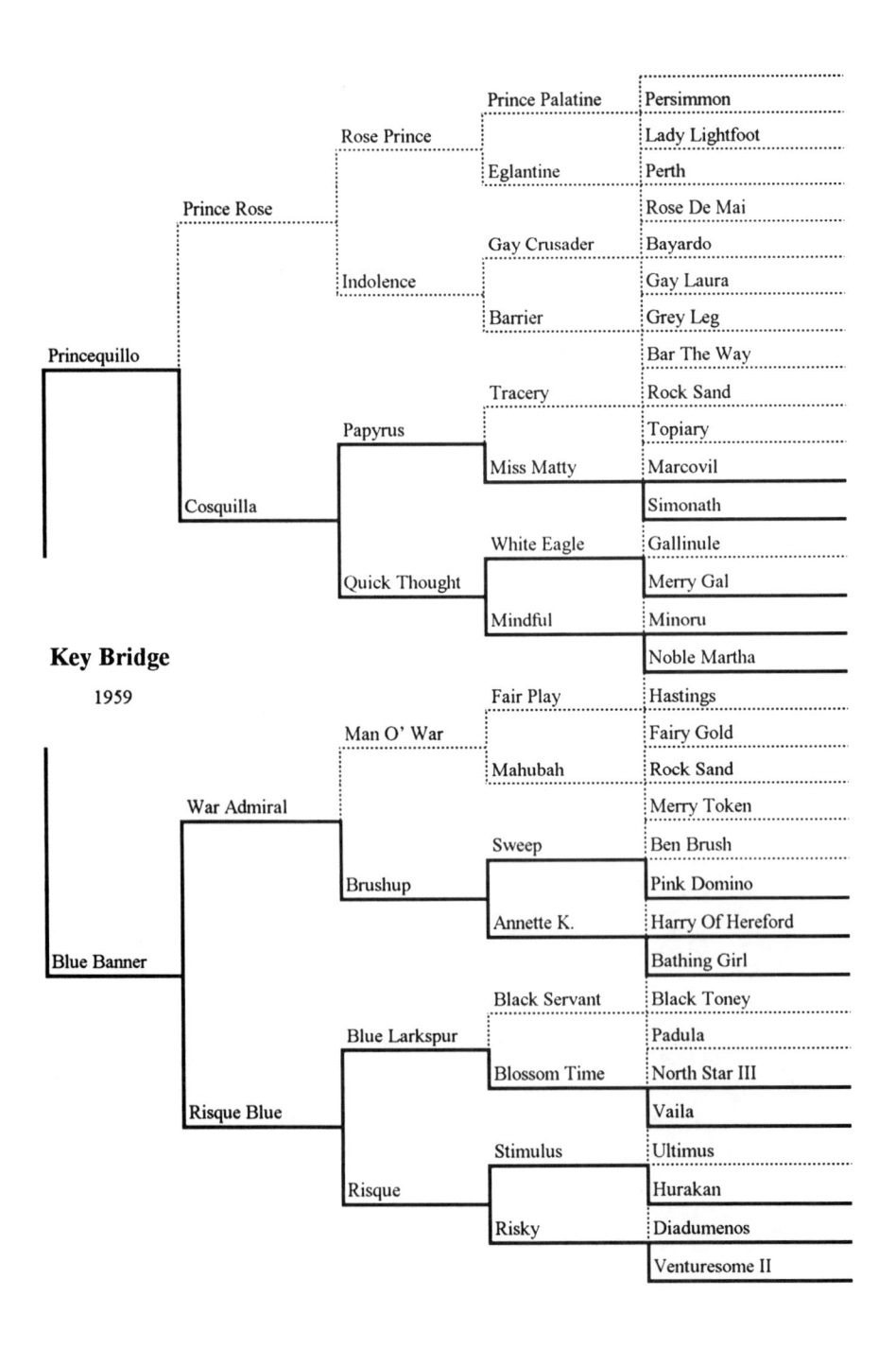

Key Bridge
1959

Pedigree

- **Princequillo**
  - Prince Rose
    - Rose Prince
      - Prince Palatine
        - Persimmon
        - Lady Lightfoot
      - Eglantine
        - Perth
        - Rose De Mai
    - Indolence
      - Gay Crusader
        - Bayardo
        - Gay Laura
      - Barrier
        - Grey Leg
        - Bar The Way
  - Cosquilla
    - Papyrus
      - Tracery
        - Rock Sand
        - Topiary
      - Miss Matty
        - Marcovil
        - Simonath
    - Quick Thought
      - White Eagle
        - Gallinule
        - Merry Gal
      - Mindful
        - Minoru
        - Noble Martha

- **Blue Banner**
  - War Admiral
    - Man O' War
      - Fair Play
        - Hastings
        - Fairy Gold
      - Mahubah
        - Rock Sand
        - Merry Token
    - Brushup
      - Sweep
        - Ben Brush
        - Pink Domino
      - Annette K.
        - Harry Of Hereford
        - Bathing Girl
  - Risque Blue
    - Blue Larkspur
      - Black Servant
        - Black Toney
        - Padula
      - Blossom Time
        - North Star III
        - Vaila
    - Risque
      - Stimulus
        - Ultimus
        - Hurakan
      - Risky
        - Diadumenos
        - Venturesome II

102

Based on performance and heart score, we know that Key to the Mint had the Princequillo heart and assume that Fort Marcy also had this heart.

Key to the Kingdom's heart, based on the identical heart scores taken of a daughter and maternal granddaughter, was probably the War Admiral heart from Key Bridge's dam. The heart scores were closely allied with the scores of the War Admiral heart size found in maternal grandsons of Buckpasser, who was out of the great War Admiral daughter, Busanda, and the My Charmer heart size found in Seattle Slew and in Desert Secret, who was her maternal grandson.

Key to the Mint's great heart, (third largest after Secretariat and Sham) was also found, intact, in his great daughter, Pure Profit, who has produced two millionaire daughters, Inside Information and Educated Risk.

Inside Information, by Private Account - another large hearted son of a Buckpasser daughter - thrilled a national audience in 1995 when she won the Breeders' Cup Distaff (G1) by 13 1/2 lengths, the largest margin of victory of any Breeders' Cup championship race ever contested since the start of the series in 1984.

Key to the Mint's great heart was present again at the 1996 Breeders' Cup when his daughter, Jewell Princess out of Jewell Ridge by Melyno (IRE), won the Breeders' Cup Distaff. The four-year-old filly has now earned more than $1.4 million. It will be interesting to see what her sons and daughters can do on the racetrack.

Another outstanding Key to the Mint daughter who inherited his large heart is Key Witness, dam of the outstanding graded stakes winners Key Contender by Fit to Fight and You'd Be Surprised by Blushing Groom.

Key Contender is currently standing at stud in New York and You'd Be Surprised produced her first foal in 1996, a colt by Seeking the Gold, another large-hearted maternal grandson of Buckpasser carrying on the War Admiral heart.

Probably the greatest of the Princequillo grandsons, in terms of heart size and performance, is Secretariat.

Secretariat's best racing offspring was his daughter, Lady's Secret, who carried his large heart to not only victory on the racetrack, but to Horse of the Year status, beating out male competitors.

Through his daughter, Weekend Surprise, multiple graded stakes winner of $402,892, Secretariat's heart found its way to grandson, A.P. Indy, who also achieved Horse of the Year status, and was a classic winner of $2,979,815. Weekend Surprise also gave Secretariat's heart to Summer Squall, another outstanding classic and multiple graded-stakes winner of more than $1.8 million.

Both of these Secretariat maternal grandsons are now producing outstanding fillies. A.P. Indy's first winner from his first crop was the filly, A.P. Assay. Summer Squall's first winners were also fillies. His daughter Storm Song, the 1996 two-year-old filly champion, won the 1996 Breeders' Cup Juvenile Fillies race at Woodbine in Toronto, Canada. She also won the Grade 1 Frizette Stakes at Belmont earlier in October. His daughter, Gale Force, won the Grade 2 Beaumont Stakes at Keeneland's spring 1996 meet in stakes-record time, in her fourth consecutive victory after five starts. His daughter, Mackie, won the Busher Handicap, and his daughter, Sugar Squeeze is stakes placed. Racing in France, his daughter, Malleret, is also stakes placed.

Secretariat's best sons, General Assembly and three-year-old champion Risen Star, had the benefit of coming from large-hearted mares. General Assembly was from a stakes-winning daughter of Native Dancer, whose heartline on his dam's tail-female line leads to his maternal great-granddam, La Chica, a daughter of Sweep, whose great heart powered War Admiral. Risen Star was out of graded-stakes winner Ribbon, by His Majesty, whose dam, Flower Bowl, was by large-hearted sire Alibhai, who traced to Pocahontas through his maternal grandsire, Tracery. Ribbon was out of a Hail to Reason daughter, Break Through. Hail to Reason's dam, Nothirdchance, was by Blue Swords, whose dam, Flaming Swords, was a daughter of the legendary large-hearted sire,

Man O' War, whose dam was out of a daughter of Sir Gallahad III, another outstanding linked sire to Pocahontas.

Terlingua, another outstanding Secretariat daughter, a multiple graded-stakes winner of $423,896, produced a leading sire in Storm Cat, winner of $570,610.

Buyers have lined up to purchase the progeny of Storm Cat, who has produced such runners as Tabasco Cat, winner of $2,347,671, out of Barbicue Sauce, by large-hearted sire Sauce Boat; Mountain Cat, out of Key to the Mint's daughter, Always Mint; and such outstanding Storm Cat daughters as: Sardula, Senate Appointee, November Snow, Stellar Cat, Missed the Storm, Caress, Desert Stormer, Tempest Dancer, Sherzarcat, OP Cat, Elrafa Ah, Joy Baby, Memories of Donny, Country Cat, Cat Attack, Ocean Cat, Cat Appeal, and Silken Cat.

In 1996, Weekend Surprise produced a very good-looking colt by Storm Cat. It will be interesting to see what this in-breeding to Secretariat and Princequillo will produce in terms of heart size and performance. On the ground, as a weanling, he looked terrific. His body type is much like that of A.P. Indy and Summer Squall, who both look very much like their dam.

Another champion maternal grandson of Secretariat, Dehere, has just had his first crop hit the ground. Dehere, out of the Secretariat daughter, Sister Dot, displayed amazing speed on the racetrack before being felled by an injury at the beginning of his third year. It will be interesting to see if his daughters live up to the promise shown by the daughters of other maternal grandsons of Secretariat.

Another proponent of the Princequillo heart, who has produced some outstanding daughters is the California-based sire Moscow Ballet, whose maternal granddam, Milan Mill, is a daughter of Princequillo. In body type, Moscow Ballet looks much like Princequillo, and in heart score, his heart is right in line with most of the Princequillo hearts. His high heart score is very close to Mill Reef's, the half-brother of his dam, Millicent.

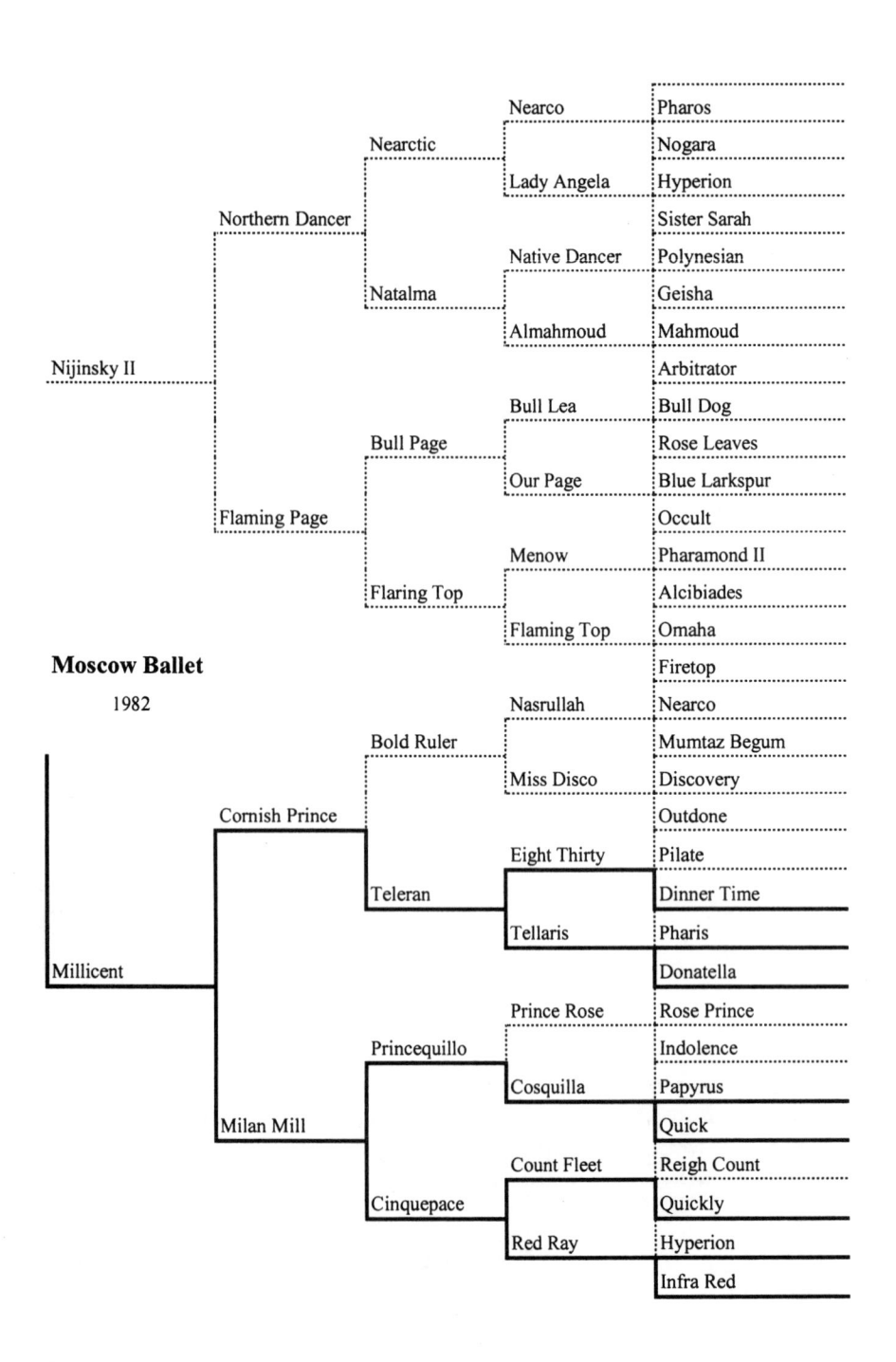

Moscow Ballet
1982

Nijinsky II
- Northern Dancer
  - Nearctic
    - Nearco
      - Pharos
      - Nogara
    - Lady Angela
      - Hyperion
      - Sister Sarah
  - Natalma
    - Native Dancer
      - Polynesian
      - Geisha
    - Almahmoud
      - Mahmoud
      - Arbitrator
- Flaming Page
  - Bull Page
    - Bull Lea
      - Bull Dog
      - Rose Leaves
    - Our Page
      - Blue Larkspur
      - Occult
  - Flaring Top
    - Menow
      - Pharamond II
      - Alcibiades
    - Flaming Top
      - Omaha
      - Firetop

Millicent
- Cornish Prince
  - Bold Ruler
    - Nasrullah
      - Nearco
      - Mumtaz Begum
    - Miss Disco
      - Discovery
      - Outdone
  - Teleran
    - Eight Thirty
      - Pilate
      - Dinner Time
    - Tellaris
      - Pharis
      - Donatella
- Milan Mill
  - Princequillo
    - Prince Rose
      - Rose Prince
      - Indolence
    - Cosquilla
      - Papyrus
      - Quick
  - Cinquepace
    - Count Fleet
      - Reigh Count
      - Quickly
    - Red Ray
      - Hyperion
      - Infra Red

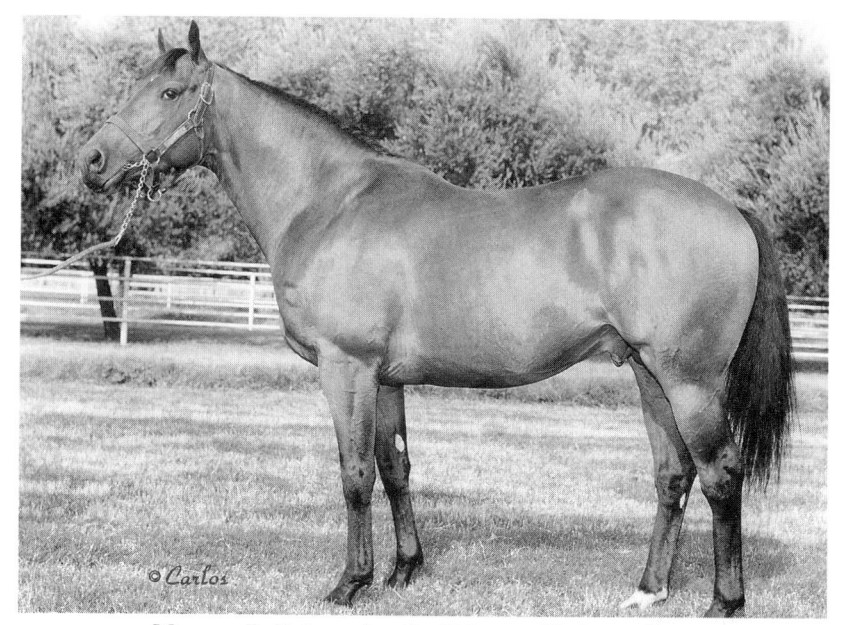

Moscow Ballet carries the Princequillo heart line

Photo by Mari Carlos
Courtesy of Harris Farms

Moscow Ballet's daughter, Soviet Problem, who inherited her sire's large heart, thrilled the world with her speed during the 1994 Breeders' Cup Sprint when she set the blazing fractions of 21.1 at the quarter, 44.3 at the half, 56.3 at the 5-furlong mark and a finish of 1:09.2, where she was caught at the wire by Cherokee Run. Soviet Problem's game race, where she led most of the way, refusing to yield in the stretch, and coming back time after time, earned her more fans than the eventual winner.

Although Soviet Problem was an outstanding sprinter, she also won the California Oaks on turf at a mile and a sixteenth. But she was happiest in sprints where her brilliant speed mowed down the competition, including two match races, one against a colt at Golden Gate Fields and another against a top stakes mare at Hollywood Park on the turf.

Earning a Beyer Speed Rating of 114 when she won the Laurel Dash (G2) in Maryland, Soviet Problem routinely turned in times of 1:08.2 for 6 furlongs in races against both colts and fillies. With earnings just under $1 million, Soviet Problem was retired after winning her first start of 1996 because of a tendon injury. She is currently in foal to Seattle Slew and should produce a large-hearted foal, whether a son or a daughter, as both the sire and the dam carry enormous hearts.

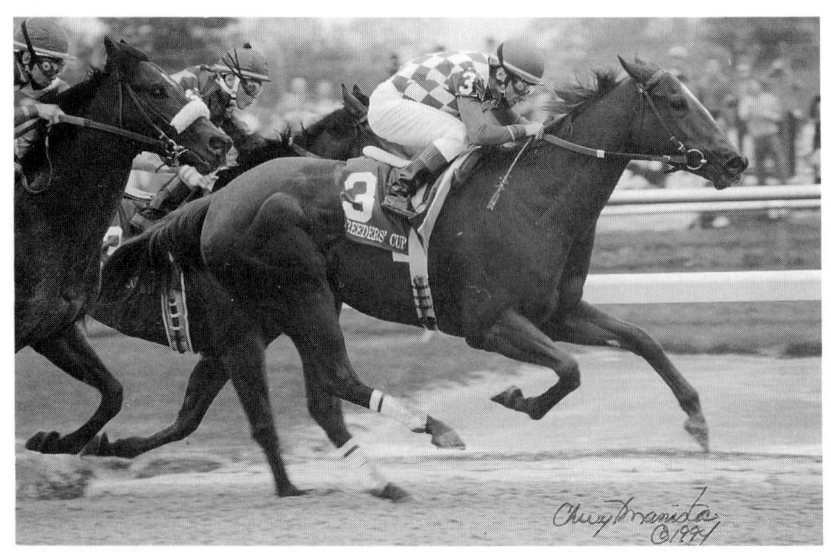

Soviet Problem set blazing fractions in the 1994 Breeders' Cup Sprint
Photo by Cheryl Manista

Two other Moscow Ballet daughters were measured in California that reflected the same large heart score. One of the mares, Moscow TV, passed on her large heart to a son, whose heart score has been measured and is currently in training..

Other large-hearted daughters of Moscow Ballet include multiple graded-stakes winner, Dominant Dancer, with earnings of $460,195; graded stakes winner Teresa Mc, with earnings of $302,945; and stakes winners Ballerina Gal, Leading Ballerina, and For My Mom.

Princequillo Heart Line Sires

A.P. Indy	Ack Ack	Afleet
Al Mamoon	Becker	Bold Bidder
Chief's Crown	Corporate Report	Danzig Connection
Defensive Play	Dehere	Diplomat Way
Dixie Brass	Dr. Blum	Farma Way
Fast Gold	Forty Niner	Gone West
Key Contender	Key to the Mint	Kris S
Mill Reef	Moscow Ballet	Mountain Cat
One For All	Pleasant Colony	Quack
Robin Des Pins	Secretariat	Sham
Sir Gaylord	Slew City Slew	Somethingfabulous
Storm Cat	Successor	Summer Squall
Sword Dance (Ire)	Tom Rolfe	

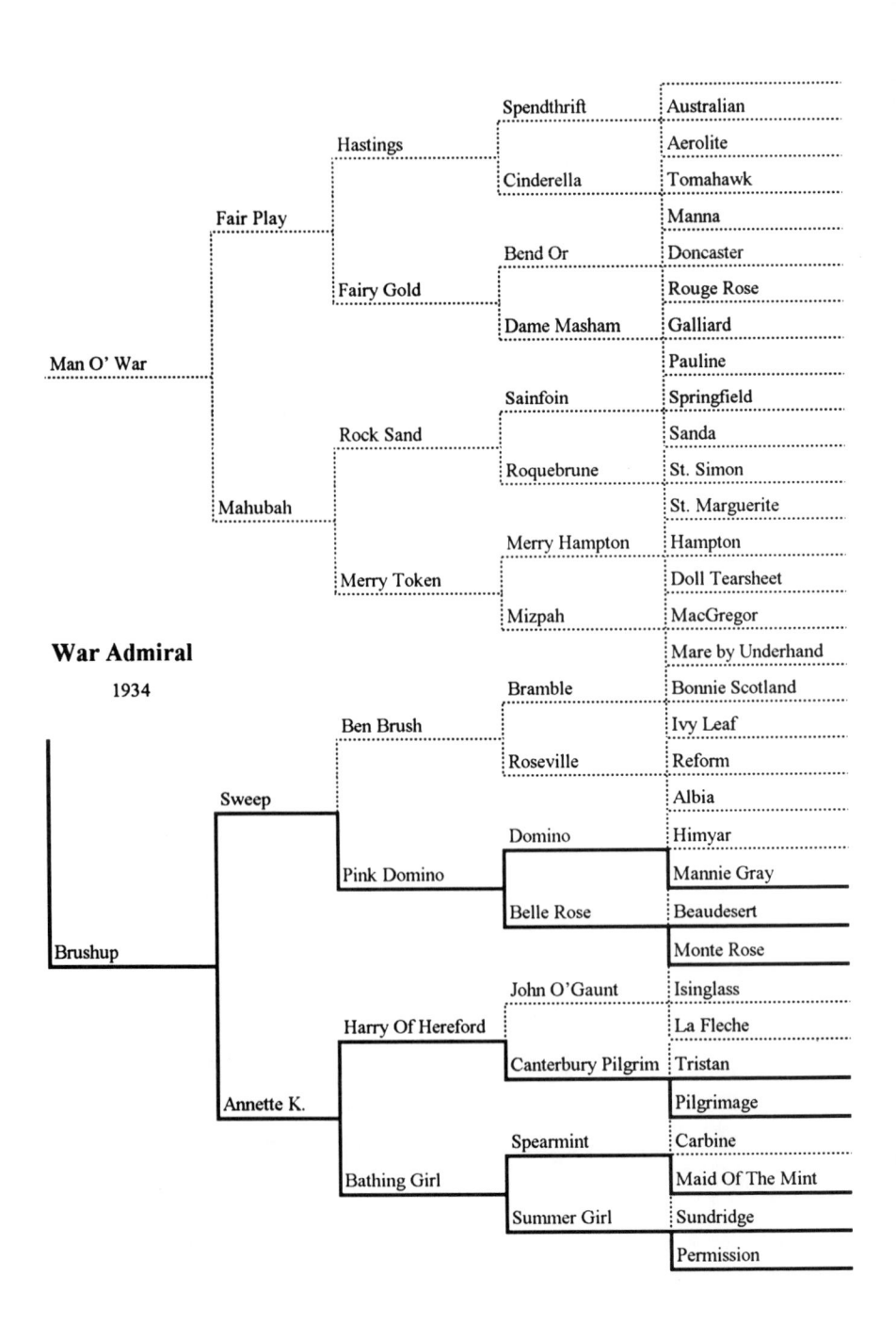

War Admiral
1934

Pedigree:

- Man O' War
  - Fair Play
    - Hastings
      - Spendthrift
        - Australian
        - Aerolite
      - Cinderella
        - Tomahawk
        - Manna
    - Fairy Gold
      - Bend Or
        - Doncaster
        - Rouge Rose
      - Dame Masham
        - Galliard
        - Pauline
  - Mahubah
    - Rock Sand
      - Sainfoin
        - Springfield
        - Sanda
      - Roquebrune
        - St. Simon
        - St. Marguerite
    - Merry Token
      - Merry Hampton
        - Hampton
        - Doll Tearsheet
      - Mizpah
        - MacGregor
        - Mare by Underhand

- Brushup
  - Sweep
    - Ben Brush
      - Bramble
        - Bonnie Scotland
        - Ivy Leaf
      - Roseville
        - Reform
        - Albia
    - Pink Domino
      - Domino
        - Himyar
        - Mannie Gray
      - Belle Rose
        - Beaudesert
        - Monte Rose
  - Annette K.
    - Harry Of Hereford
      - John O'Gaunt
        - Isinglass
        - La Fleche
      - Canterbury Pilgrim
        - Tristan
        - Pilgrimage
    - Bathing Girl
      - Spearmint
        - Carbine
        - Maid Of The Mint
      - Summer Girl
        - Sundridge
        - Permission

110

Chapter 14

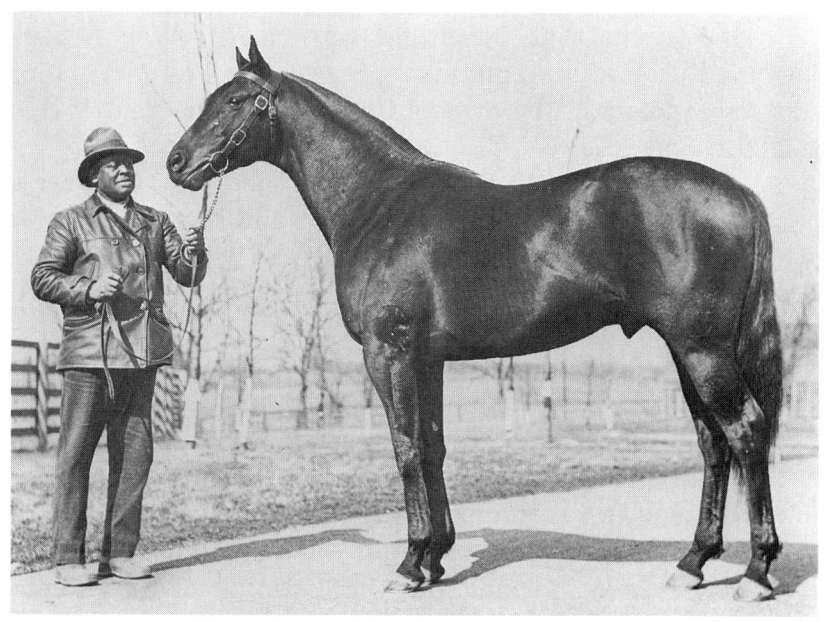

War Admiral

War Admiral (Man O' War x Brush Up)
Photo courtesy of the Keeneland Library

War Admiral's great heart came from his dam, Brush Up, a double copy mare by the outstanding sire and broodmare sire, Sweep, who was out of Pink Domino by Domino, and traced back along the X chromosome line to Pocahontas. Another Sweep daughter, Dustwhirl, produced Whirlaway. Whirlaway's heart line can be found on the X-chromosome line in the sire, Bet Twice.

Sweep was another case of a small horse with a big heart. He had speed and a hardy constitution, winning nine of 13 starts and never being out of the money. He won the 1909 Futurity, National Stallion, Belmont and Carlton Stakes, and the Lawrence Realization. His best daughters were Brush Up and Dustwhirl, both producing champions.

War Admiral's daughter, Busher, Horse of the Year in 1945, has a doubling up of Sweep in her pedigree. Her dam, Baby League, was by Bubbling Over who was out of a Sweep mare, Beaming Beauty.

It is said that, when he was racing, War Admiral resembled his maternal grandsire, Sweep. War Admiral's large heart races today in the mighty Cigar, out of the Seattle Slew daughter, Solar Slew.

Seattle Slew's dam, My Charmer, had War Admiral on the X chromosome line on both her top and bottom. Her sire, Poker, was a maternal grandson of the War Admiral daughter, Striking, and her maternal grandsire, Jet Action was out of the great War Admiral daughter, Busher.

In addition to carrying on in the Seattle Slew daughters, War Admiral is represented in all the maternal grandsons of Buckpasser. Buckpasser was out of Busanda, by War Admiral out of Businesslike by Blue Larkspur.

Some of the outstanding large-hearted sires represented by this War Admiral-Blue Larkspur cross found in Buckpasser daughters include: Seeking the Gold, winner of $2.3 million and sire of the champion fillies Flanders and Heavenly Prize; Woodman, Irish champion 2-year-old, and sire of such daughters as graded stakes winners, Gay Gallanta, Kathie's Colleen, Andromaque, Wood of Binn, Genovefa, and Bosra Sham; English and Irish champion El Gran Senor, winner of $520,969, and sire of such daughters as Irish champion Flowing and multiple stakes winners, Bright Candles, Toussaud, Crystal Gazing, Corrazona, Navarra, and Chanzi; and Private Account, winner of $339,396 and sire of undefeated champion Personal Ensign, winner of more than $1.6 million, and dam of millionaire daughter My Flag, by another Buckpasser maternal grandson, champion Easy Goer, winner of more than $4.8 million.

Dr. Fager, the first and only horse to be awarded all the titles for which he was eligible - Horse of the Year, champion sprinter, champion handicap horse, and champion grass horse - also ran on the War Admiral heart, courtesy of his dam, Aspidistra, by Better Self, who was out of Bee Mac, a daughter of War Admiral. Aspidistra also gave that heart to her daughter, champion Ta Wee, who passed it on to her offspring, like Great Above and Entropy.

Following the pattern found in large-hearted sires, Dr. Fager became known as a sire of fillies and an outstanding broodmare sire. He sired Dearly Precious, champion two-year-old filly, and Canadian Horse of the Year, L'Alezane, a leading distaff performer and multiple stakes winner of more than $367,000.

His daughter, Killaloe, who also carried the heart line of Princequillo, through her maternal granddam, Cequillo, a daughter of Princequillo, passed on her large heart to her son, Fappiano, who was an outstanding sire of sons and daughters. Fappiano is the broodmare sire of the champion two-year-old filly, Storm Song, a daughter of Summer Squall out of Hum Along by Fappiano. Her pedigree indicates that she is a probable double copy for the large-heart characteristic.

When Killaloe died at the end of September, 1996, her autopsy revealed that she had a very large heart consistent with the War Admiral heart size. This means that she expressed her sire's heart and carried the Princequillo heart on her other X chromosome, making her a double copy mare.

When bred to large-hearted mares, like Gana Facil, who was tail-female to Dr. Fager's dam, Aspidistra, through her maternal granddam, Magic, a daughter of Buckpasser, Fappiano sired sons like Kentucky Derby winner, Unbridled, winner of more than $4.4 million, and Cahill Road, Grade I stakes winner of $370,280. When bred to Naval Orange, whose sire Hoist the Flag, was out of the War Admiral daughter, Wavy Navy, and whose dam, Mock Orange, was out of the Blue

Larkspur daughter, Alablue, he sired Cryptoclearance, winner of more than $3.7 million.

Cryptoclearance has continued the pattern of the large-hearted sire by siring daughters like Strategic Maneuver.

Dr. Fager's daughter, Quick Cure, produced the sire, Cure the Blues, who is following the pattern, also. When bred to mares with large-heart lines, he gets successful sons like Lucratif, champion three-year-old colt in Italy, who was out of a daughter of large-hearted sire, Mill Reef.

As time goes on, daughters by Cure the Blues, Cryptoclearance, Cahill Road, and Unbridled will become more and more valuable, just as daughters of the other large-hearted lines will as they pass the characteristic on to their offspring.

Some of the other outstanding broodmare sires and young sires carrying the War Admiral heart are:

War Admiral Heart Line Sires

Academy Award	Affirmed	Allen's Prospect.
Alysheba	Believe It	Bet Twice
Better Self	Broad Brush	Buckpasser
Bupers	Cahill Road	Crafty Admiral
Cryptoclearance	Cure the Blues	Desert Secret
Dr. Fager	Easy Goer	El Gran Senor
Fappiano	Fast Play	Great Above
Hoist The Flag	Housebuster	Irish Open
Lomond	Mining	Personal Flag
Plugged Nickle	Private Account	Quiet American
Rare Performer	Seattle Slew	Seeking the Gold
Silent Screen	Swaps	Sweep
Wavering Monarch	Whirlaway	With Approval
Woodman		

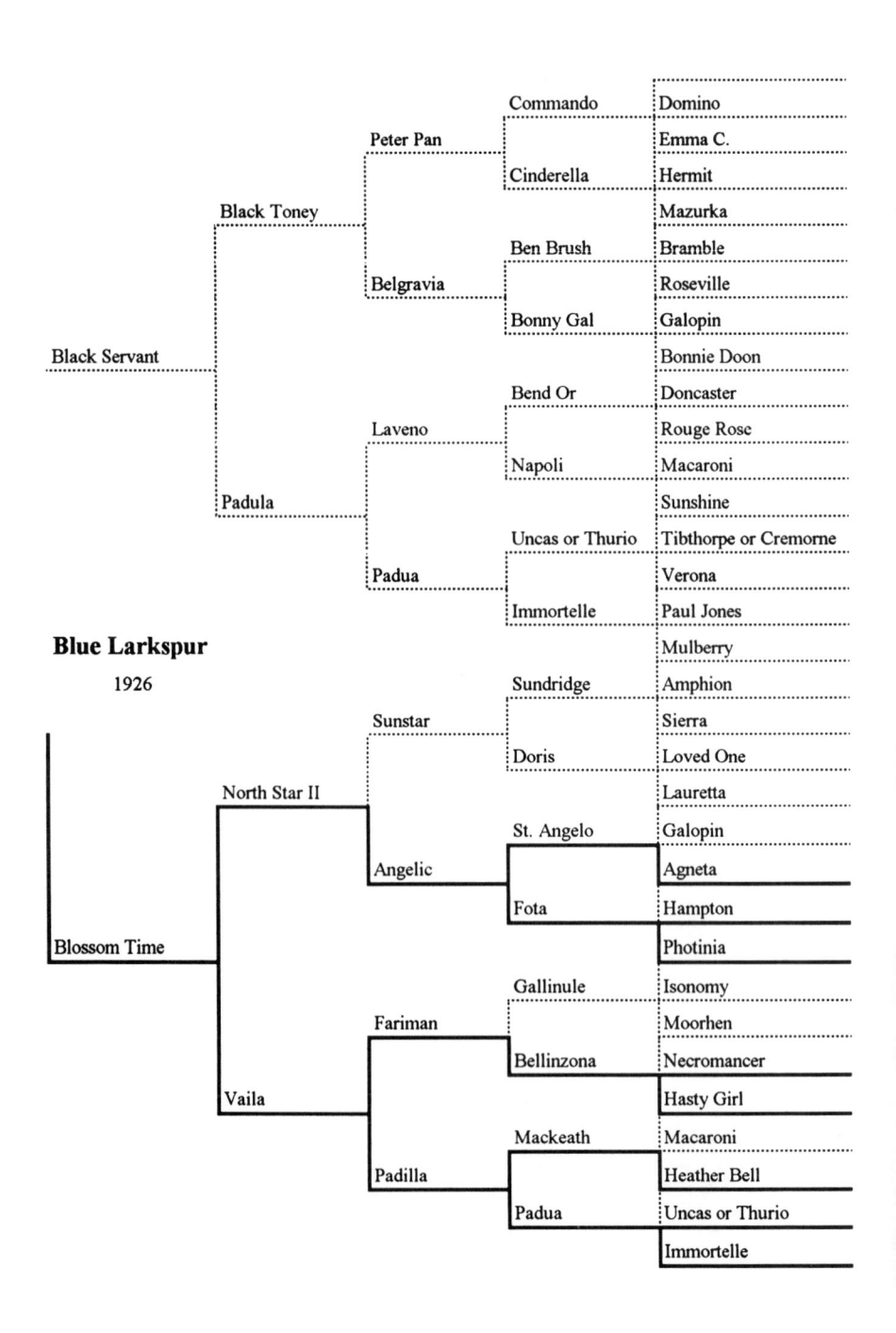

Blue Larkspur
1926

- Black Servant
  - Black Toney
    - Peter Pan
      - Commando
        - Domino
        - Emma C.
      - Cinderella
        - Hermit
        - Mazurka
    - Belgravia
      - Ben Brush
        - Bramble
        - Roseville
      - Bonny Gal
        - Galopin
        - Bonnie Doon
  - Padula
    - Laveno
      - Bend Or
        - Doncaster
        - Rouge Rose
      - Napoli
        - Macaroni
        - Sunshine
    - Padua
      - Uncas or Thurio
        - Tibthorpe or Cremorne
        - Verona
      - Immortelle
        - Paul Jones
        - Mulberry

- Blossom Time
  - North Star II
    - Sunstar
      - Sundridge
        - Amphion
        - Sierra
      - Doris
        - Loved One
        - Lauretta
    - Angelic
      - St. Angelo
        - Galopin
        - Agneta
      - Fota
        - Hampton
        - Photinia
  - Vaila
    - Fariman
      - Gallinule
        - Isonomy
        - Moorhen
      - Bellinzona
        - Necromancer
        - Hasty Girl
    - Padilla
      - Mackeath
        - Macaroni
        - Heather Bell
      - Padua
        - Uncas or Thurio
        - Immortelle

Chapter 15

Blue Larkspur

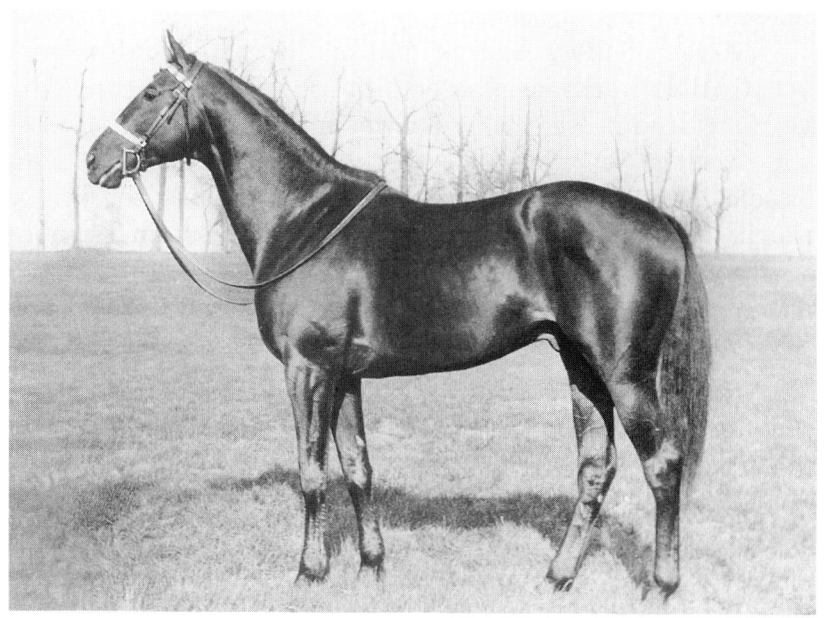

Blue Larkspur (Black Servant x Blossom Time)
Photo courtesy of Grayson / Sutcliffe Collection

Blue Larkspur will long be remembered for his daughters who have kept his heart alive today through horses like Nijinsky II, Roberto, Green Dancer, Boldnesian, Alydar, Bates Motel, Damascus, Fly So Free, Riverman, Dayjur, Smile, Slewpy, Prince John, Personal Hope, Stalwart, Alydeed, Batonnier, Red Ransom, Skywalker, Relaunch, Cohoes, Little Missouri, Caveat, Mr. Prospector, Blushing John, Big Spruce, Alleged, Bold Reason, T.V. Lark, Zanthe, and Devil's Bag.

When Blue Larkspur daughters were bred to War Admiral and the resulting foal was a filly, the mating produced mares like Busanda, dam of Buckpasser, who has had a profound effect on large-hearted maternal grandsons. Another outstanding combination was that of War Admiral with the Blue Larkspur daughter, Risque Blue, which produced the stakes-winning mare, Blue Banner. Blue Banner produced the 1980 Broodmare of the Year, Key Bridge, who gave the Princequillo heart to sons Key to the Mint and Fort Marcy and the Blue Larkspur - War Admiral heart to son Key to the Kingdom and Key to Content.

A son of Black Servant out of Blossom Time by North Star III, Blue Larkspur was bred by Edward Riley Bradley at Idle Hour Stud in Kentucky. He was a solid bay, short-backed, with excellent shoulders, withers, and gaskins. His dam, Blossom Time was a good race mare at 2, winning the Pimlico Futurity, Brilliance and Consolation Stakes. Blossom Time was out of a mare Bradley purchased in England in 1915, Vaila, by Fariman out of Padilla. Bradley paid approximately $400. She was quite a bargain.

Blue Larkspur, racing from 1928 through 1930, won 10 of 16 starts and earned $272,070, a considerable amount at that time. Among the stakes he won were the Juvenile, National Stallion, Saratoga Special, Withers, Belmont, Classic, Stars and Stripes Handicap and the Arlington Cup.

Blue Larkspur had many great daughters who went on to influence the breed through their sons and daughters, such as: Lady Lark (dam of champion Twilight Tear, 1944's Horse of the Year); Our Page, dam of sire Bull Page, who sired Nijinsky II's dam, Flaming Page; Light Lark (maternal great granddam of T.V. Lark); Banish Fear (dam of Cosmic Bomb, broodmare sire of Halo, and maternal granddam of Prince John); Blue Delight (dam of champion filly, Real Delight, maternal granddam of Sweet Tooth, dam of Alydar); Businesslike (dam of Busanda, dam of Buckpasser); Alablue (maternal granddam of Boldnesian); multiple stakes winner Elpis (maternal great granddam of Go Step); Blue Denim (maternal great granddam of Grey Dawn II); and Bloodroot (dam of Bimlette and multiple stakes winner, Be Faithful, granddam of Bold Reason).

One of his greatest daughters may have been the great race mare, Myrtlewood, dam of Miss Dogwood, who is the dam of Sequence, the dam of Gold Digger, who is the dam of Mr. Prospector. Myrtlewood is also the maternal granddam of Myrtle Charm, dam of Fair Charmer, who is the dam of My Charmer, the dam of Seattle Slew.

Blue Larkspur Heart Line Sires

Alleged	Alydar	Alydeed
Bates Motel	Batonnier	Big Spruce
Blushing John	Bold Reason	Boldnesian
Buckpasser	Caveat	Cohoes
Damascus	Dayjur	Devil's Bag
Fly So Free	Green Dancer	Grey Dawn II
Halo	Little Missouri	Mr. Prospector
Nijinsky II	Personal Hope	Prince John
Red Ransom	Relaunch	Riverman
Roberto	Seattle Slew	Skywalker
Slewpy	Smile	Stalwart
T.V. Lark	Zanthe	

Mahmoud
1933

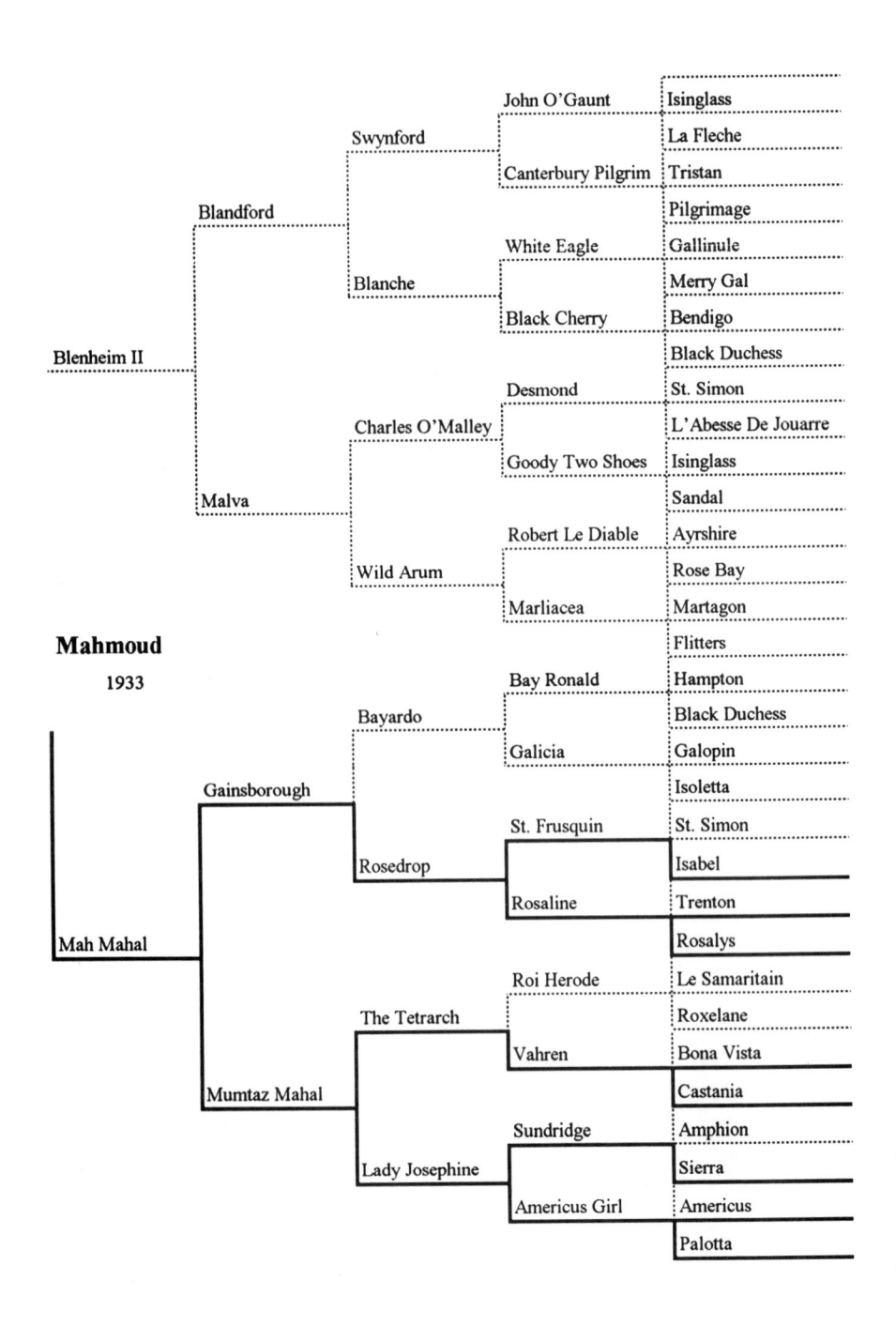

Blenheim II	Blandford	Swynford	John O'Gaunt	Isinglass
				La Fleche
			Canterbury Pilgrim	Tristan
				Pilgrimage
		Blanche	White Eagle	Gallinule
				Merry Gal
			Black Cherry	Bendigo
				Black Duchess
	Malva	Charles O'Malley	Desmond	St. Simon
				L'Abesse De Jouarre
			Goody Two Shoes	Isinglass
				Sandal
		Wild Arum	Robert Le Diable	Ayrshire
				Rose Bay
			Marliacea	Martagon
				Flitters
Mah Mahal	Gainsborough	Bayardo	Bay Ronald	Hampton
				Black Duchess
			Galicia	Galopin
				Isoletta
		Rosedrop	St. Frusquin	St. Simon
				Isabel
			Rosaline	Trenton
				Rosalys
	Mumtaz Mahal	The Tetrarch	Roi Herode	Le Samaritain
				Roxelane
			Vahren	Bona Vista
				Castania
		Lady Josephine	Sundridge	Amphion
				Sierra
			Americus Girl	Americus
				Palotta

Chapter 16

Mahmoud

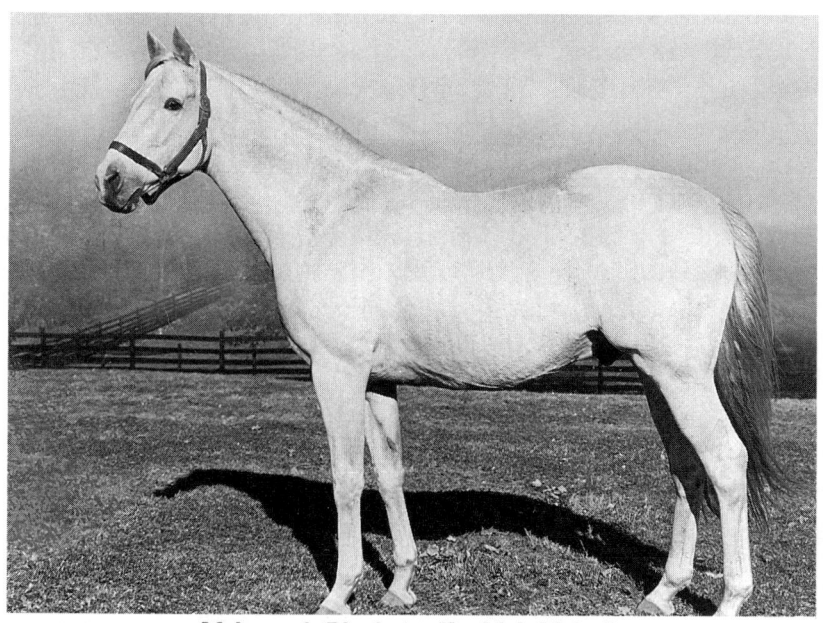

Mahmoud (Blenheim II x Mah Mahal)
Photo courtesy of the Keeneland Library

English champion Mahmoud, winner of the 1936 Epsom Derby, was by Blenheim II out of Mah Mahal, whose dam, Mumtaz Mahal, was the granddam of Nasrullah. A beautiful gray, almost white, stallion, Mahmoud stood 15.2-3/4 hands high. He was the first foal from his dam, Mah Mahal, who was by Gainsborough out of the fleet Mumtaz Mahal. He was foaled in the spring of 1933. As a two-year-old, he won the Exeter Stakes at Newmarket, the Richmond Stakes at Goodwood and the Champagne Stakes at the St. Leger meeting in the fall of 1935 at Doncaster.

Mahmoud won only one race as a three-year-old, but it was a good one - the English Derby. Ironically, he won by three lengths in record time of 2:33-4/5, lowering the time of another large-hearted sire, Hyperion, who had established the previous Derby record of 2:34 in 1933.

This great sire and broodmare sire gave his large heart to the likes of Northern Dancer, Gallant Man, Holy Bull, Halo, His Majesty, Rahy, Demons' Begone, Graustark, Majestic Prince, Mickey McGuire, Grey Dawn II, Spectacular Bid, Skip Trial, Silver Ghost, Sir Harry Lewis, Risen Star, Opening Verse, Pine Bluff, Flying Continental, Waquoit, State Dinner, Sovereign Dancer, Rainbows For Life, Tasso, Homebuilder, What A Pleasure, and Arazi.

Mahmoud's pedigree is closely allied to that of Nasrullah, another large-hearted sire. They both share the same maternal granddam, Mumtaz Mahal. During his four years at stud in Ireland, Mahmoud followed the pattern of large-hearted sires with his best offspring being daughters. During that time, he sired Irish Guiness and Oaks winner Majideh, who passed on his large heart to her daughter, English Oaks winner Masaka and her son, Belmont Stakes winner, Gallant Man; and Donatella III, the best two-year-old of her year in Italy and the dam of eight stakes winners in England and Italy.

C. V. Whitney bought Mahmoud for approximately $85,000 in 1940 and brought him to Kentucky where he was a great success at stud. He died at the age of 29 at the Whitney Farm in 1962.

Among the outstanding daughters he sired who have gone on to pass on his large heart are: champion First Flight; Almahmoud, dam of Natalma, dam of Northern Dancer; Grey Flight, dam of nine stakes winners, including champion Misty Morn.

A large-hearted daughter of Mickey McGuire, who is carrying the Mahmoud heart was measured during the study.

This stakes-winning daughter, Shayne McGuire, had a very large heart, with a heart score of 137, that she has passed along to her graded and multiple stakes winning daughter, Teresa Mc, winner of $302,945. Theresa Mc, when measured, was found to have a heart score of 137-140. Shayne McGuire's stakes-winning three-year-old son, Mr. Thrifty, was also measured and found to have a heart score of 147-150. This score is consistent with the Mahmoud heart size found in Northern Dancer. Shayne McGuire has done very well when crossed with the large-hearted sire, Moscow Ballet.

Northern Dancer, who has the large heart of Mahmoud, passed it along to his daughters, who in turn passed it to their progeny, like Arazi, who has been measured and found to have a very large heart consistent with the size of Northern Dancer. In the project, the large Mahmoud heart was found in Northern Dancer daughters. Northern Dancer had an ECG taken of his heart when he was 23 that revealed he had a very large heart, with a heart score of 150, consistent with the size found in his daughters and other Mahmoud descendants on the X-chromosome lines.

Size has not been found to be a factor in the large heart. The biggest hearts are not necessarily found in the biggest horses. Mill Reef was only 15.2 hands, yet he had a heart that was twice the normal size. Moscow Ballet is only 15.3, yet he has a very large heart with a heart score of 147. His paternal grandsire, Northern Dancer, was a small stallion who stood 15.3. He had a tremendous impact on the breed, and he was measured and found to have a very large heart score of 150.

Mahmoud Heart Line Stallions

Arazi	Demons' Begone	Flying Continental	Gallant Man
Graustark	Grey Dawn II	Halo	His Majesty
Holy Bull	Homebuilder	Majestic Prince	Mickey McGuire
Northern Dancer	Opening Verse	Pine Bluff	Rahy
Rainbows For Life	Risen Star	Silver Ghost	Sir Harry Lewis
Skip Trial	Sovereign Dancer	Spectacular Bid	State Dinner
Tasso	Waquoit	What A Pleasure	

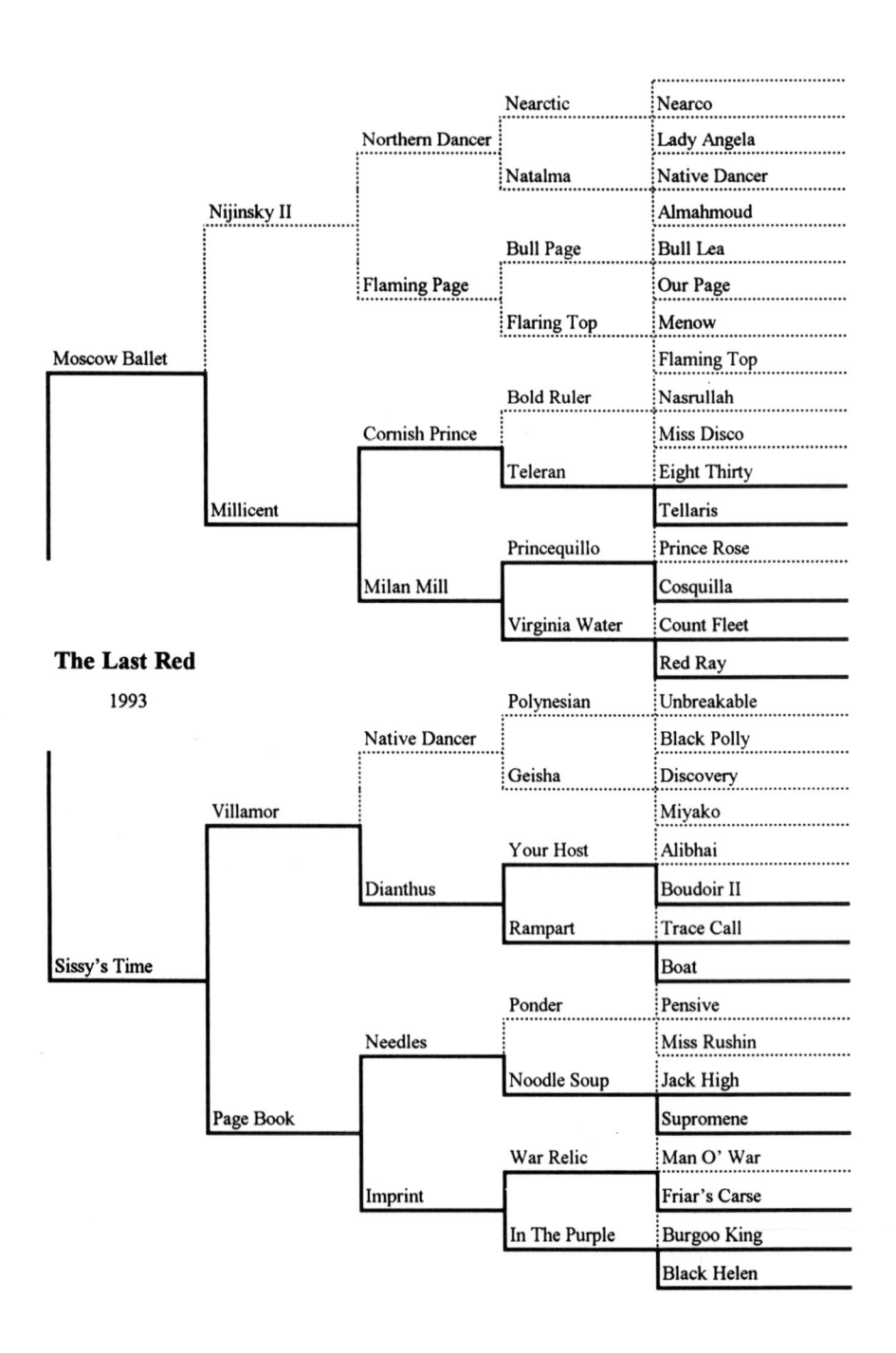

The Last Red
1993

- Moscow Ballet
  - Nijinsky II
    - Northern Dancer
      - Nearctic
        - Nearco
        - Lady Angela
      - Natalma
        - Native Dancer
        - Almahmoud
    - Flaming Page
      - Bull Page
        - Bull Lea
        - Our Page
      - Flaring Top
        - Menow
        - Flaming Top
  - Millicent
    - Cornish Prince
      - Bold Ruler
        - Nasrullah
        - Miss Disco
      - Teleran
        - Eight Thirty
        - Tellaris
    - Milan Mill
      - Princequillo
        - Prince Rose
        - Cosquilla
      - Virginia Water
        - Count Fleet
        - Red Ray

- Sissy's Time
  - Villamor
    - Native Dancer
      - Polynesian
        - Unbreakable
        - Black Polly
      - Geisha
        - Discovery
        - Miyako
    - Dianthus
      - Your Host
        - Alibhai
        - Boudoir II
      - Rampart
        - Trace Call
        - Boat
  - Page Book
    - Needles
      - Ponder
        - Pensive
        - Miss Rushin
      - Noodle Soup
        - Jack High
        - Supromene
    - Imprint
      - War Relic
        - Man O' War
        - Friar's Carse
      - In The Purple
        - Burgoo King
        - Black Helen

Chapter 17

Large Hearts in Small Packages

Large hearts can come in very small packages. Moscow Ballet also gave his large heart to a tiny twin filly, The Last Red. She weighed only 52 pounds at birth, compared to the 102 pounds of her brother. She was a surprise at foaling, having not shown up on an early ultrasound.

Upon examination of the placenta after her birth, it was found that she had only 30% attachment to the placenta, giving her only one-third the nutrients that her twin brother received during gestation.

But the tiny twin, who only needed some oxygen and heart massage and was on her feet on the second day with no extraordinary help, was raised along with her brother, Check Off Dollars, by her dam, Sissy's Time. When running in the field with her larger sibling, she could run rings around him even though she was little more than half his size.

Because we were able to measure both her sire and her dam, we found that the twin filly had the same large heart size consistent with the Princequillo heart. Her dam, Sissy's Time, a multiple and graded-stakes winner, had a large heart as well, with a heart score of 127-130, but it was significantly smaller than her tiny daughter's, whose heart score was 140.

Her twin brother, who was carrying the mother's heart, went off to the races at two and broke his maiden on his second start by 8 1/2 lengths at Golden Gate Fields in California. He won again at three, going wire to wire in the mud at Bay

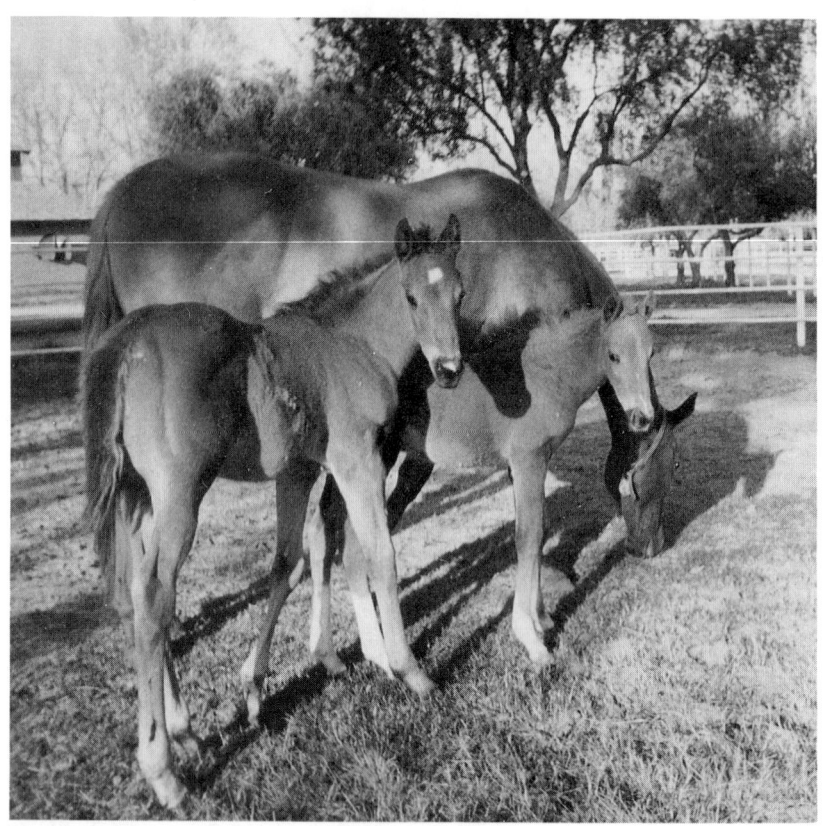

The Last Red shown with her twin brother, Check Off Dollars. Because of her large heart, she is participating in a breeding experiment in Kentucky.

Photo courtesy of Harris Farm

Meadows. This is unusual for a twin and he didn't even have the biggest heart.

At 3, the twin filly stood 14.3 and had a heart as large as some champion stallions. When she was shipped into Kentucky, it was noticed that she had a beautiful stride and a lot of speed. But, as she had come to Kentucky to participate in a breeding experiment on the large heart and there were no 3/4-size jockeys around, that speed and heart will have to go on to the next generation.

Because we knew the size of both her sire and dam's heart, and because of the heart lines in her pedigree, we were

Whirlaway
1938

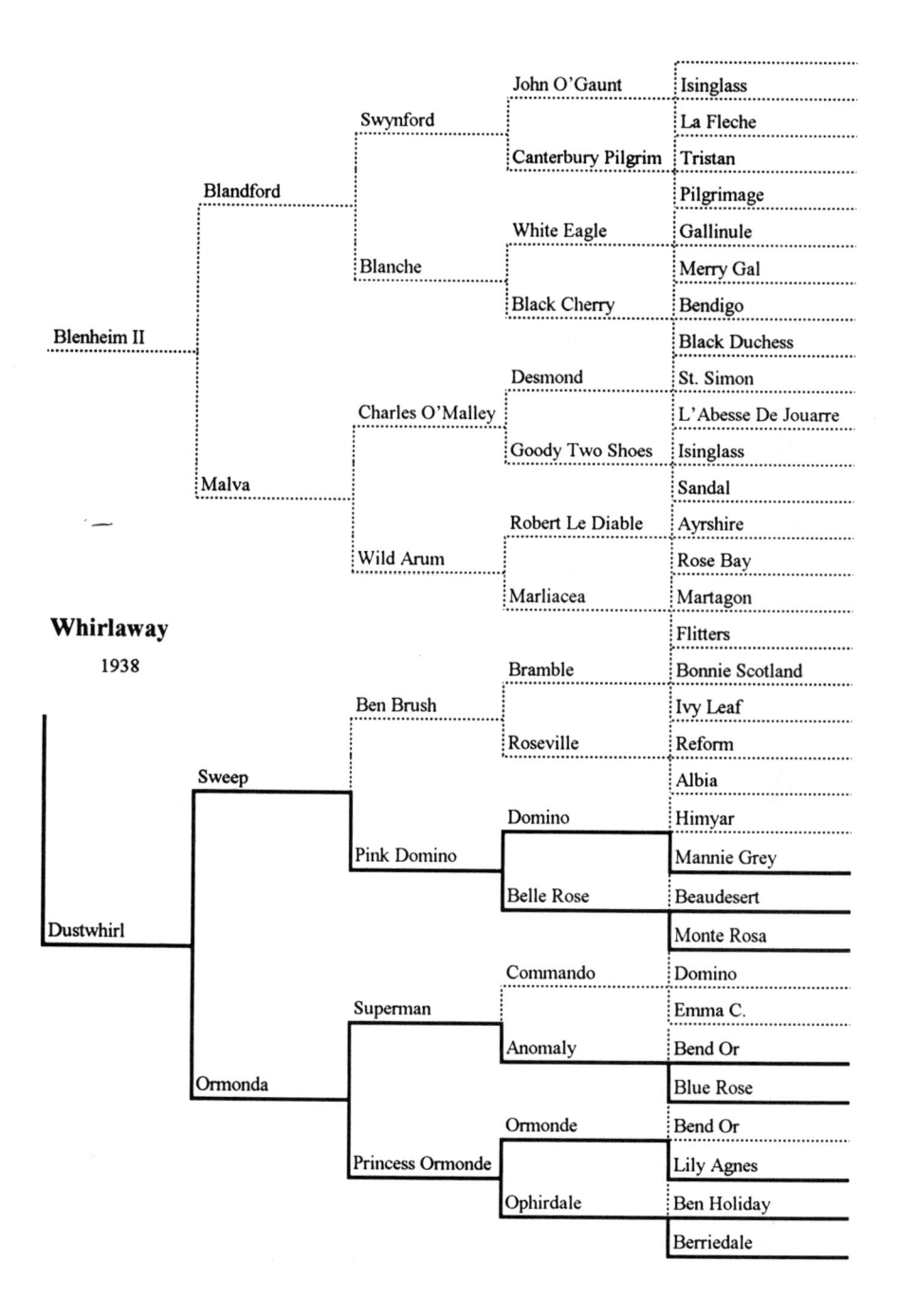

Blenheim II	Blandford	Swynford	John O'Gaunt	Isinglass
				La Fleche
			Canterbury Pilgrim	Tristan
				Pilgrimage
		Blanche	White Eagle	Gallinule
				Merry Gal
			Black Cherry	Bendigo
				Black Duchess
	Malva	Charles O'Malley	Desmond	St. Simon
				L'Abesse De Jouarre
			Goody Two Shoes	Isinglass
				Sandal
		Wild Arum	Robert Le Diable	Ayrshire
				Rose Bay
			Marliacea	Martagon
				Flitters
Dustwhirl	Sweep	Ben Brush	Bramble	Bonnie Scotland
				Ivy Leaf
			Roseville	Reform
				Albia
		Pink Domino	Domino	Himyar
				Mannie Grey
			Belle Rose	Beaudesert
				Monte Rosa
	Ormonda	Superman	Commando	Domino
				Emma C.
			Anomaly	Bend Or
				Blue Rose
		Princess Ormonde	Ormonde	Bend Or
				Lily Agnes
			Ophirdale	Ben Holiday
				Berriedale

able to determine that the twin filly was probably homozygous for the large heart characteristic, or what we call a "double copy." That means she carries her mother's heart on one X and her sire's heart on the other.

What we found as we have tracked the inheritance of the characteristic supports the idea that the genetic trait is co-dominant. Given this supposition, because the twin filly carries her sire's heart, that means she carries the large heart on both of her X chromosomes. This makes her a double copy, capable of passing on the large heart to all of her offspring.

As part of the on-going project, the twin filly has been bred to a large-hearted stallion, Desert Secret. Desert Secret has a fascinating bottom side for the large-hearted characteristic. He is out of a daughter of Secretariat who was out of My Charmer, the dam of another large-hearted sire, Seattle Slew, the leading broodmare sire of 1995.

When Desert Secret was measured, he was found to have a very large heart, with a heart score of 140, which is consistent with the War Admiral heart size found in the Seattle Slew line. That told us that the X chromosome he got from his dam, Clandestina, was the one she got from her dam, My Charmer, dam of Seattle Slew.

Although The Last Red is a twin, her size is based on the lack of nutrition she received while inside her dam because of the 30 percent attachment to the placenta. While small, she is perfectly conformed with a deep girth, a wasp waist, and a long underline which gives her an amazing stride and considerable speed. Because of these attributes, she has earned the stable name of "Mighty Mouse." Although she is physically small, genetically she will reproduce normal-sized offspring.

It was because of her size, her large heart, and her pedigree that she was selected to be used for a test breeding of this characteristic.

Based on what we have learned following the inheritance patterns of this characteristic, if The Last Red produces a colt, it should have either Sissy's Time's heart or Moscow Ballet's heart or a combination of the two. If she has a filly, it should have a choice of three heart sizes, including Desert Secret's large heart.

The large heart has not always been a blessing. If everything else works well, it has enabled some horses to rise above the herd and thrill the world with their speed. But when that race record is not followed by famous sons of these racing champions, their stock in the breeding shed falls rapidly and the spotlight is quickly turned off. The lack of understanding that some of their best attributes - such as large heart size - may have been sex-linked led to an early fall from grace which was only stopped years later when their daughters began to produce sons that could win.

History is littered with such horses as Whirlaway, Citation, and Omaha, who performed amazing feats on the racetrack and were later deemed unworthy as sires because they were unable to pass on their greatness to sons. It is interesting to note the large heart lines in their pedigrees. Omaha was 4x4 to Pocahontas. Citation was out of a daughter of Hyperion, a legendary large-hearted broodmare sire. Whirlaway was out of Dust Whirl by Sweep, the same large-hearted line that gave War Admiral his large heart.

The only remembrance of these great stallions is through their daughters. Omaha's great heart passed down through his maternal grandson Summer Tan and is found in the modern pedigrees of Air Forbes One, Proud Truth, Full Pocket, Slewacide, Ivatan, champion Top Knight, out of his maternal granddaughter, Ran-Tan, Lord Durham (sire of Canadian champion fillies, Choral Group and Stage Flite) and Orbit's Scene. Omaha's heart line is also in Nijinsky II's pedigree through his daughter, Flaming Top, the maternal granddam of Nijinsky II's dam, Flaming Page.

Citation sired the champion filly Silver Spoon, who is the maternal granddam of Grade 1 winner and sire, Coined Silver and the graded stakes winning sire, Metfield. Citation also has his heart line in Afleet's pedigree through his daughter, Piccalili.

Whirlaway sends his heart down the X-chromosome trail through his daughter, Whirla Lea, on the tail-female line of the sire Bet Twice, winner of more than $3.3-million.

PART V

PUTTING THE X FACTOR TO WORK

Chapter 18

Covering the Genetic Bases

In measuring heart scores, doing pedigree research, and checking autopsy reports of some of yesterday's and today's greatest sires and dams as well as examining horses currently in training and failed racehorses, it has been possible to identify the largest heart lines found in today's breeding stock, all tracing back to Eclipse on the X chromosome line through the mare, Pocahontas. This is important knowledge to have when engaged in breeding outstanding athletes because of the pattern of performance found in the large-hearted individuals. But there are pitfalls ahead.

When it comes to the genetic recipe for a large heart in a racehorse, the way can become tricky because of the possible combinations on the genetic wheel of fortune. Breeding a colt is easier, of course, since the only concern is the bottom side of the pedigree for the large-heart characteristic. But, as only God gets to decide the sex of the offspring, the breeder must plan each mating for every contingency.

That means a breeder needs a large-hearted sire in case the resulting foal is a filly and inherits her dominant X chromosome from her sire. A breeder also has to make sure the sire has an outstanding top line to take care of whatever comes down the Y chromosome that he passes on to his son. The breeder then looks at the dam's pedigree to ensure that all the elements for success are available no matter which of the two X chromosomes on the dam's pedigree comes into play in forming the new racehorse.

Bold Ruler
1954

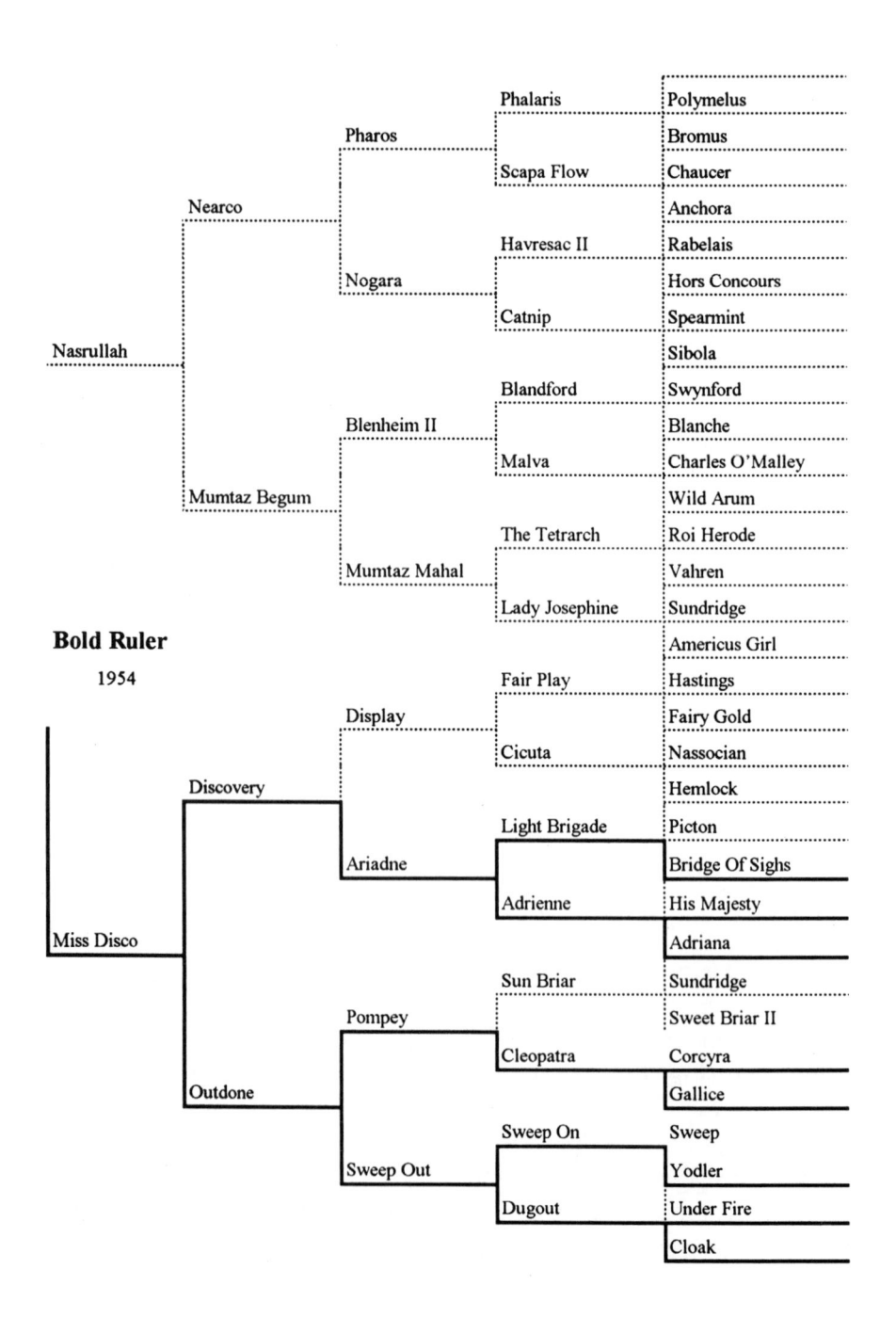

- Nasrullah
  - Nearco
    - Pharos
      - Phalaris
        - Polymelus
        - Bromus
      - Scapa Flow
        - Chaucer
        - Anchora
    - Nogara
      - Havresac II
        - Rabelais
        - Hors Concours
      - Catnip
        - Spearmint
        - Sibola
  - Mumtaz Begum
    - Blenheim II
      - Blandford
        - Swynford
        - Blanche
      - Malva
        - Charles O'Malley
        - Wild Arum
    - Mumtaz Mahal
      - The Tetrarch
        - Roi Herode
        - Vahren
      - Lady Josephine
        - Sundridge
        - Americus Girl

- Miss Disco
  - Discovery
    - Display
      - Fair Play
        - Hastings
        - Fairy Gold
      - Cicuta
        - Nassocian
        - Hemlock
    - Ariadne
      - Light Brigade
        - Picton
        - Bridge Of Sighs
      - Adrienne
        - His Majesty
        - Adriana
  - Outdone
    - Pompey
      - Sun Briar
        - Sundridge
        - Sweet Briar II
      - Cleopatra
        - Corcyra
        - Gallice
    - Sweep Out
      - Sweep On
        - Sweep
        - Yodler
      - Dugout
        - Under Fire
        - Cloak

This is especially important if the resulting foal is a colt since he will only inherit an X chromosome from his dam and he has a 50-50 chance of getting either her top or bottom side. If the resultant foal is a filly, it is even more complicated because she will have a choice of three X chromosomes - one from her sire and one of two from her dam. There is no way to know which X chromosome will be dominant and thus expressed, so it is important to make sure that all three choices are the best available.

For centuries, top breeders have followed the axiom of breeding the best to the best. Because of the relationship between the large heart and a pattern of performance, this tradition has enabled the large heart to race down countless generations leaping from top mare to son to daughter to daughter and son and so on.

But because there is no understanding of the relationship of a large heart to the accomplishments of an outstanding colt the breeding can be hit or miss. Such was the case with Whirlaway. When he was not bred to a correspondingly large-hearted mare, he was unable to reproduce anything close to himself in a son.

Even with his daughters, if the dam had a normal-sized heart, his daughter may not have expressed his heart size and wouldn't be recognized for some years until she produced a colt or a daughter that received and expressed the large-hearted X chromosome the dam had inherited from her sire.

The Thoroughbred breeding industry is always looking for instant gratification. For centuries, greatness in a sire has only been recognized through the sire's sons. There is only a secondary recognition for sires who produce outstanding daughters. But the real glory has been reserved for the sire of sires. In light of what has been discovered about what has really powered many of the mighty stallions, it is ironic that what really made those sons great was not their sires, but their dams.

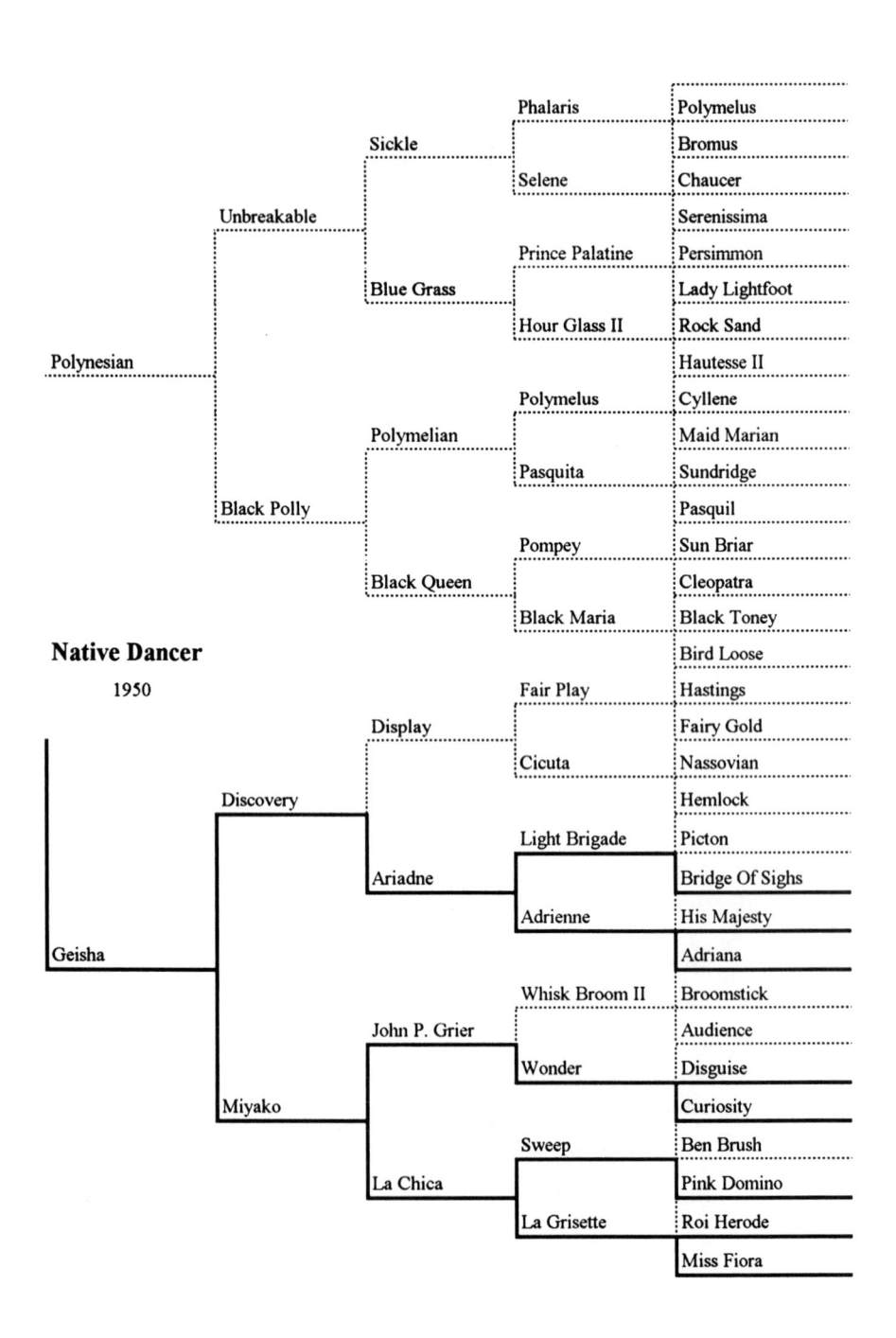

Native Dancer
1950
Polynesian
Unbreakable
Sickle
Phalaris
Polymelus
Bromus
Selene
Chaucer
Serenissima
Blue Grass
Prince Palatine
Persimmon
Lady Lightfoot
Hour Glass II
Rock Sand
Hautesse II
Black Polly
Polymelian
Polymelus
Cyllene
Maid Marian
Pasquita
Sundridge
Pasquil
Black Queen
Pompey
Sun Briar
Cleopatra
Black Maria
Black Toney
Bird Loose
Geisha
Discovery
Display
Fair Play
Hastings
Fairy Gold
Cicuta
Nassovian
Hemlock
Ariadne
Light Brigade
Picton
Bridge Of Sighs
Adrienne
His Majesty
Adriana
Miyako
John P. Grier
Whisk Broom II
Broomstick
Audience
Wonder
Disguise
Curiosity
La Chica
Sweep
Ben Brush
Pink Domino
La Grisette
Roi Herode
Miss Fiora

Bold Ruler's best son, Secretariat, raced on a mighty heart courtesy of his dam, Somethingroyal. Before Secretariat was sired, the word on Bold Ruler was that he couldn't sire a colt that could stay the distance. Then came Secretariat. With his large heart's oxygen pumping ability, distance wasn't a problem, and coupled with his mighty stride, he amazed the world in his 31-length victory in the mile-and-a-half Belmont Stakes.

With the hindsight of autopsy reports, an interesting circumstance is observed in comparing the pedigree of Bold Ruler, who had a normal-sized heart with that of Native Dancer, who ended up producing some outstanding daughters who passed on large hearts to their progeny.

Both stallions were out of daughters of Discovery, but it is the bottom side of their dam's pedigree that tells the story.

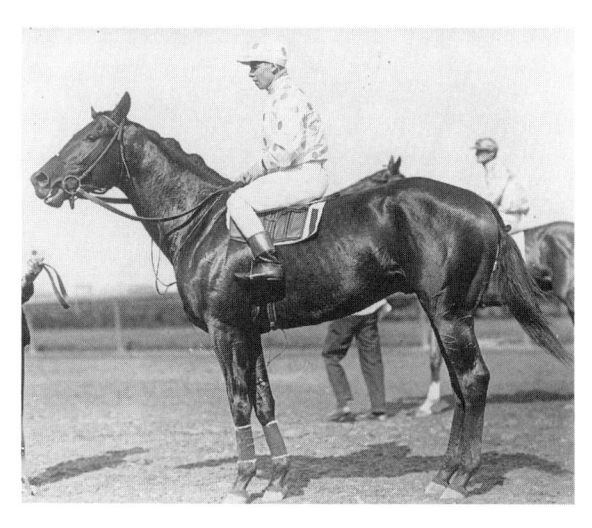

Sweep 1907
(Ben Brush x Pink Domino)

Sweep's large-hearted daughters produced War Admiral and Whirlaway

Photo courtesy of the Keeneland Library

Native Dancer's dam, Geisha, on the tail-female line, was the granddaughter of a daughter of Sweep, who has an outstanding large heart line to Pocahontas through Stockwell's daughter, Woodbine. Sweep daughters produced War Admiral, Whirlaway, and Bubbling Over, all of whom passed on their large hearts through their daughters.

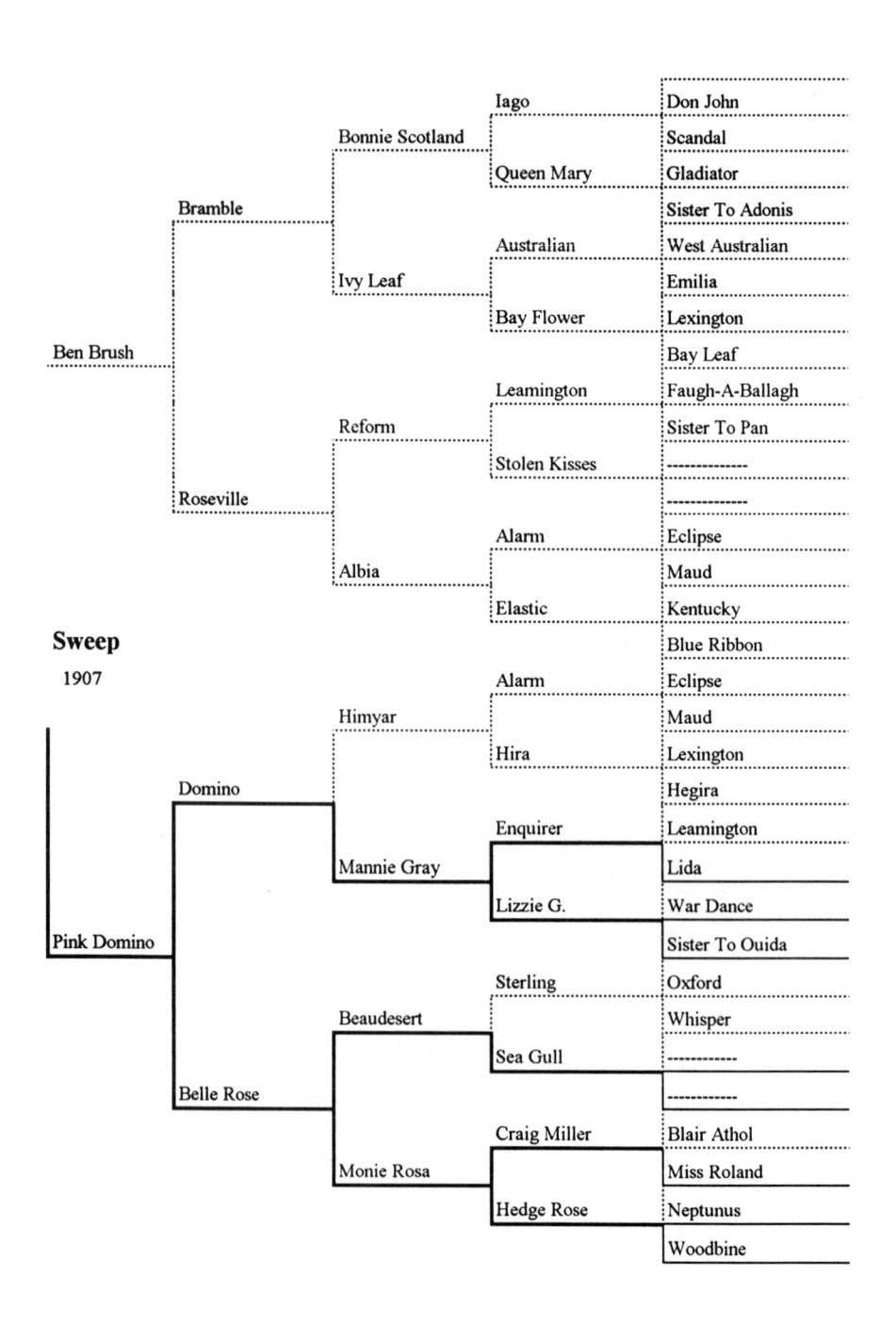

Sweep
1907

Ben Brush	Bramble	Bonnie Scotland	Iago	Don John
				Scandal
			Queen Mary	Gladiator
				Sister To Adonis
		Ivy Leaf	Australian	West Australian
				Emilia
			Bay Flower	Lexington
				Bay Leaf
	Roseville	Reform	Leamington	Faugh-A-Ballagh
				Sister To Pan
			Stolen Kisses	------------

		Albia	Alarm	Eclipse
				Maud
			Elastic	Kentucky
				Blue Ribbon
Pink Domino	Domino	Himyar	Alarm	Eclipse
				Maud
			Hira	Lexington
				Hegira
		Mannie Gray	Enquirer	Leamington
				Lida
			Lizzie G.	War Dance
				Sister To Ouida
	Belle Rose	Beaudesert	Sterling	Oxford
				Whisper
			Sea Gull	------------

		Monie Rosa	Craig Miller	Blair Athol
				Miss Roland
			Hedge Rose	Neptunus
				Woodbine

On the other hand, Bold Ruler's dam, Miss Disco, on the tail-female line, was a granddaughter of a daughter of Sweep's son, Sweep On, who could not inherit Sweep's large heart, as he only inherited a Y chromosome from his sire. Bold Ruler, like other sires of sires is fading from pedigrees, with dwindling tail-male influence, but Native Dancer, like other outstanding broodmare sires, will live on due to their influence on the X chromosome.

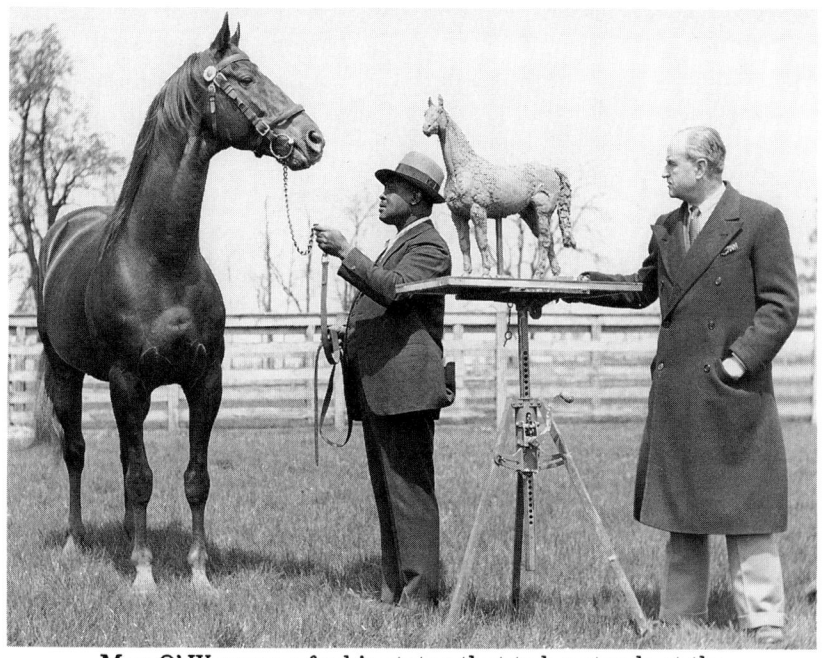

Man O' War poses for his statue that today stands at the Kentucky Horse Park, Lexington, KY.
Photo courtesy of the Grayson/Sutcliffe Collection

Man O' War's greatest son, War Admiral, won the Triple Crown with the help of a heart inherited from his dam, Brushup. War Admiral took after his maternal grandsire, Sweep, being a small brown horse rather than a large golden chestnut like his sire, Man O' War. Following the pattern of the X-Factor line, War Admiral became an amazing broodmare sire but was considered a failure as a sire of sires.

Man O' War
1917

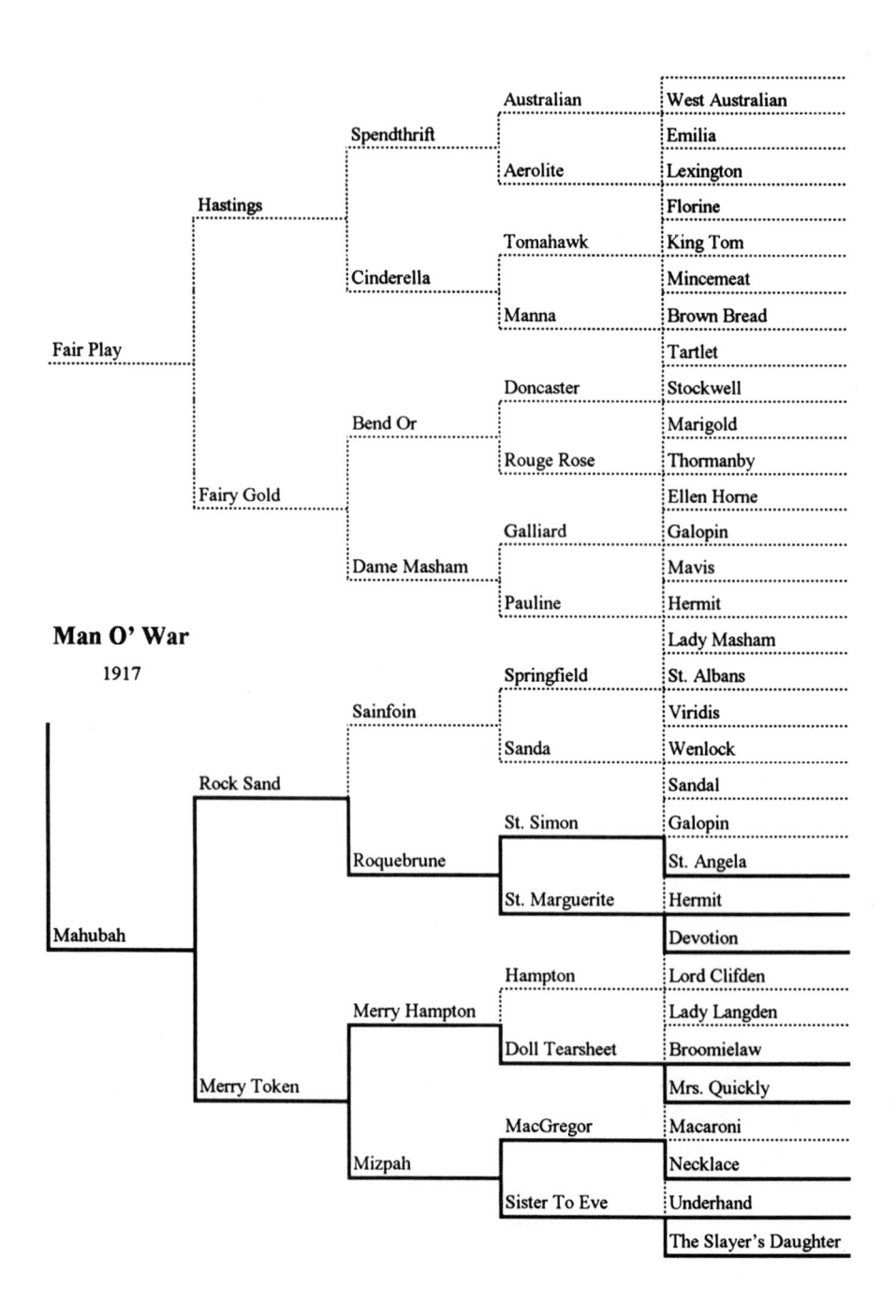

Fair Play	Hastings	Spendthrift	Australian	West Australian
				Emilia
			Aerolite	Lexington
				Florine
		Cinderella	Tomahawk	King Tom
				Mincemeat
			Manna	Brown Bread
				Tartlet
	Fairy Gold	Bend Or	Doncaster	Stockwell
				Marigold
			Rouge Rose	Thormanby
				Ellen Horne
		Dame Masham	Galliard	Galopin
				Mavis
			Pauline	Hermit
				Lady Masham
Mahubah	Rock Sand	Sainfoin	Springfield	St. Albans
				Viridis
			Sanda	Wenlock
				Sandal
		Roquebrune	St. Simon	Galopin
				St. Angela
			St. Marguerite	Hermit
				Devotion
	Merry Token	Merry Hampton	Hampton	Lord Clifden
				Lady Langden
			Doll Tearsheet	Broomielaw
				Mrs. Quickly
		Mizpah	MacGregor	Macaroni
				Necklace
			Sister To Eve	Underhand
				The Slayer's Daughter

This shows how foolish is the idea that only a sire of sires can be considered brilliant. Very little passes on the Y chromosome and after 50 years, there is nothing but "paper potency" left in direct male descendants. But War Admiral's heart races today in horses like Cigar and in all the female progeny of stallions like Woodman, Seattle Slew, Private Account, El Gran Senor, With Approval, Seeking the Gold, Desert Secret, and Dr. Fager, not to mention the progeny of their daughters. He will live in pedigrees for generations after all those sires of sires like Bold Ruler have faded from the scene.

Man O' War, through his maternal grandsire, Rock Sand, had an outstanding large-heart line to Pocahontas. Rock Sand's dam, Roquebrune was a daughter of the great sire and broodmare sire, St. Simon, whose dam, St. Angela, was a daughter of Pocahontas' son, King Tom. His maternal great-granddam, Devotion, on the tail-female line, was a daughter of Pocahontas' son, Stockwell.

Thanks to that large heart line, Man O' War was among the 10 leading broodmare sires for 22 years. Because of the large heart he inherited from his maternal grandsire, Rock Sand, Man O' War not only demonstrated a legendary pattern of performance, but he also followed the same pattern of other large-hearted sires on the Pocahontas heart line such as Stockwell, King Tom, Rataplan, St. Simon, Wellingtonia, John O'Gaunt, Isonomy, Roi Herod, Ajax, Chaucer, Phalaris, Gainsborough, Sundridge, Isinglas, Bend Or, and Sainfoin.

Rock Sand was another outstanding racehorse, winning the English Triple Crown in 1903. When he was bred to the mare, Topiary, who had Pocahontas on the top and bottom of her pedigree through her paternal great-granddam, St. Angela, by King Tom and her maternal grandsire, Wellingtonia, out of Pocahontas' daughter, Araucaria, the resulting foal was the outstanding sire, Tracery. Tracery would go on to sire some outstanding daughters who would pass the Pocahontas heart on to sires like Alibhai.

Rock Sand
1900

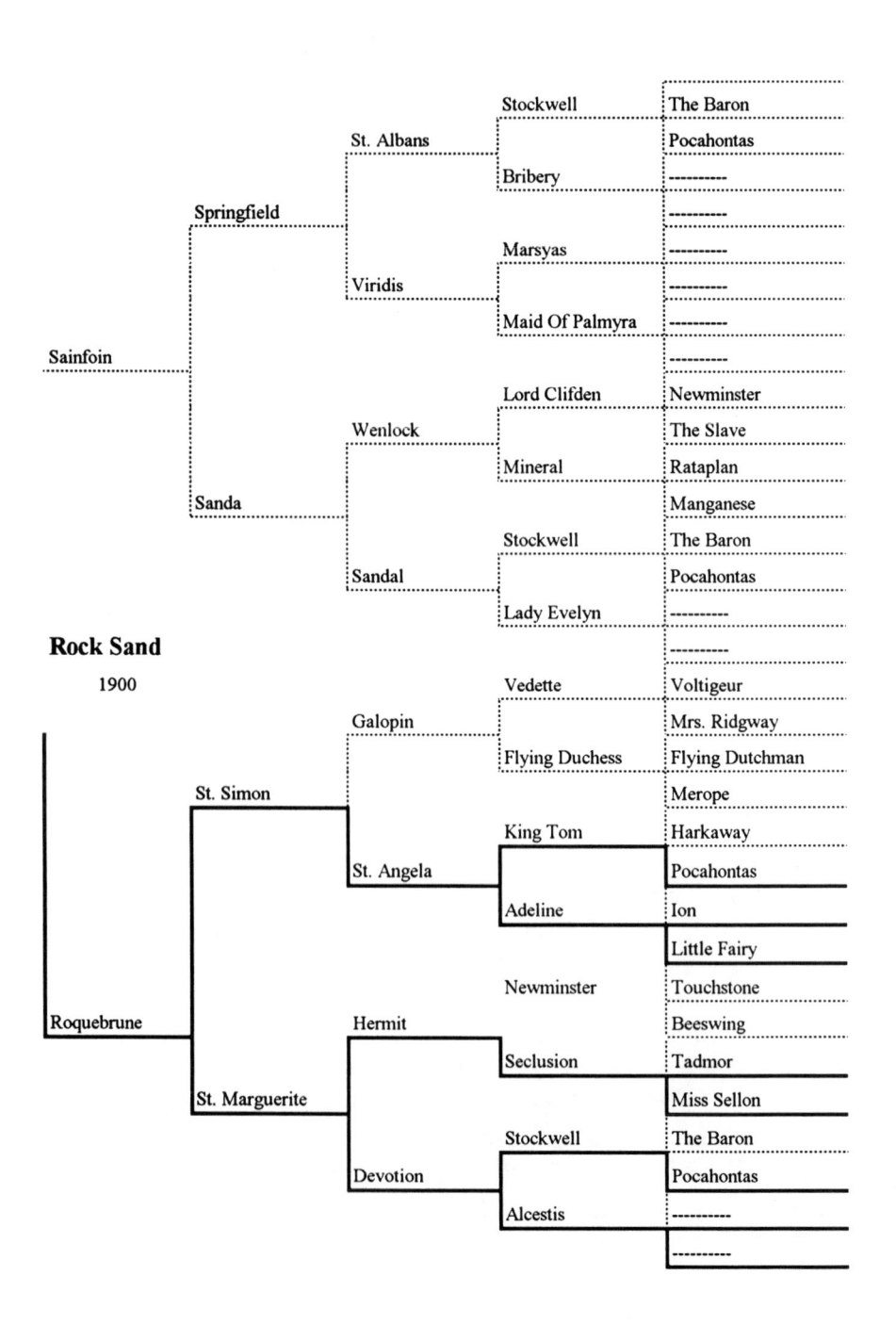

Sainfoin	Springfield	St. Albans	Stockwell	The Baron
				Pocahontas
			Bribery	----------

		Viridis	Marsyas	----------

			Maid Of Palmyra	----------

	Sanda	Wenlock	Lord Clifden	Newminster
				The Slave
			Mineral	Rataplan
				Manganese
		Sandal	Stockwell	The Baron
				Pocahontas
			Lady Evelyn	----------

Roquebrune	St. Simon	Galopin	Vedette	Voltigeur
				Mrs. Ridgway
			Flying Duchess	Flying Dutchman
				Merope
		St. Angela	King Tom	Harkaway
				Pocahontas
			Adeline	Ion
				Little Fairy
	St. Marguerite	Hermit	Newminster	Touchstone
				Beeswing
			Seclusion	Tadmor
				Miss Sellon
		Devotion	Stockwell	The Baron
				Pocahontas
			Alcestis	----------

142

Alibhai would, in turn, produce daughters like champion Bornastar, Flower Bowl, dam of Graustark, who would continue the X Factor line through his daughters, and champion Bowl of Flowers. Although he never raced, Alibhai's autopsy would reveal he had a large heart near the size of the great heart of Eclipse.

Rock Sand's heart would also be present in the tail-female line of Count Fleet's dam, Quickly, through her granddam, Malachite, a daughter of Rock Sand.

Man O' War's great heartline is found in the pedigree of the sire, Eight Thirty, whose dam, Dinner Time was out of Man O' War's daughter, Seaplane. Eight Thirty is a name found frequently on the X chromosome line of large-hearted horses.

That great dam, Plucky Liege, who produced six stakes-winning sons, of which three were classic winners and four became leading sires, was out of a daughter of St. Simon, Concertina, connecting her to Pocahontas on the X chromosome through St. Angela, by King Tom. Four of Plucky Liege's sons, Sir Gallahad III, Bull Dog, Admiral Drake, and Bois Roussel, became leading broodmare sires in England, France, and North America.

Sir Gallahad III's daughters produced a total of 139 stakes winners including Challedon, another large-heart line sire. His son Roman, who sired the later-day Pocahontas, linked up to the original Pocahontas on his dam's side through his granddam, Look Up, a daughter of Ultimus out of the Sweep daughter, Sweeping Glance.

Those "failed" sires of sires like War Admiral, Blue Larkspur, Buckpasser, and Secretariat, will live on long after those other "better" sires of sires have disappeared into the dust of time.

What has been learned is still an unfolding story. The pedigree research has shown not only that all the large heart line stallions became broodmare sires and tracked on the X chromosome line to Eclipse through Pocahontas, but that there seemed to be a similarity in body type associated with the large-heart line. It is not only the Princequillo heart-line horses that look alike.

War Admiral was said to resemble his maternal grandsire, Sweep. Hyperion more closely resembled his dam, Selene and her sire, Chaucer; taking his color from Chaucer's dam, Canterbury Pilgrimage, another horse linked to Pocahontas on the heart line.

Further research may reveal a link between the large-heart gene and body type on the X chromosome. It is not inconceivable given what we see in photographic comparisons of horses linked on the X chromosome and current research into human body types and what they can mean in terms of inheritable diseases. If heart size can be linked to body type, then heart conditions may be linked to inheritable body types in humans on the X chromosome. This could give scientists a better indicator of what to watch for in human patients.

Understanding the difference between no copy, a single copy, and double-copy individuals in the area of large hearts in racehorses is important. The most important thing that should be done with a prospective mare is to have her heart measured, whether with an ECG or the use of ultrasound.

A mare with no copy would have a normal sized heart and no heart lines on the X chromosome lines of her pedigree. This mare would be unable to pass on the large heart to her offspring, with the exception of a daughter that got her dominant X chromosome from a large-hearted sire.

A single copy mare may or may not express the large heart, but has the ability to pass it on to 50 percent of her progeny.

A double copy mare would have the large-heart trait on both of her X chromosomes and would pass it on to all of her progeny. In the case of daughters, if mated to a large-hearted sire, she would produce double copy daughters as well. This is what happened with Secretariat's daughter, Weekend Surprise, whose dam, Lassie Dear was also a double copy. Lassie Dear was a daughter of the outstanding broodmare sire, Buckpasser, and out of a daughter of Sir Gaylord, out of

Somethingroyal, a daughter of Princequillo and the dam of Secretariat.

Another double copy mare is Hopespringseternal, the dam of the large-hearted sire, Miswaki. Hopespringseternal is by Buckpasser out of a daughter of Princequillo, with her tail-female line going to a daughter of Nasrullah out of a daughter of Bull Lea.

With Hopespringset___ ___ds lead to Pocahontas. Three of the four larg___ ___es are represented in her pedigree, with a conn___ ___ fourth, Mahmoud, through Nasrullah, who ha___ ___e maternal granddam as Mahmoud. A daugh___ ___opespringseternal was measured and found to have a heart score of 147.

The double copy mares are highly prized because they have a pattern of producing practically all winners and many outstanding individuals, such as Lassie Dear did with Weekend Surprise and Wolfhound, and Weekend Surprise did with A.P. Indy and Summer Squall.

This information gathered from either an ECG or an ultrasound, coupled with an in-depth pedigree of at least five generations, is important in establishing where the mare is in regards to this inheritable trait. Until the genetic marker is found, which will make it a matter of a simple blood test, this is the best way to know what you are dealing with in trying to breed a top performance athlete.

Since it is the mare that passes on this trait to her sons and to 50 percent of her daughters, she is the most important one to measure. Certain heart lines are very consistent as long as they are in the proper part of the pedigree.

When looking at a mare's pedigree, a breeder must look at the bottom side of her sire's pedigree, specifically his dam's pedigree, checking her sire and her dam, paternal granddam, and maternal granddam and grandsire, zigzagging backward on the dam's side, always following the X chromosome trail which goes from sire to daughter to daughter and son. When going backward through a pedigree it is sire to dam to

Halo

1969

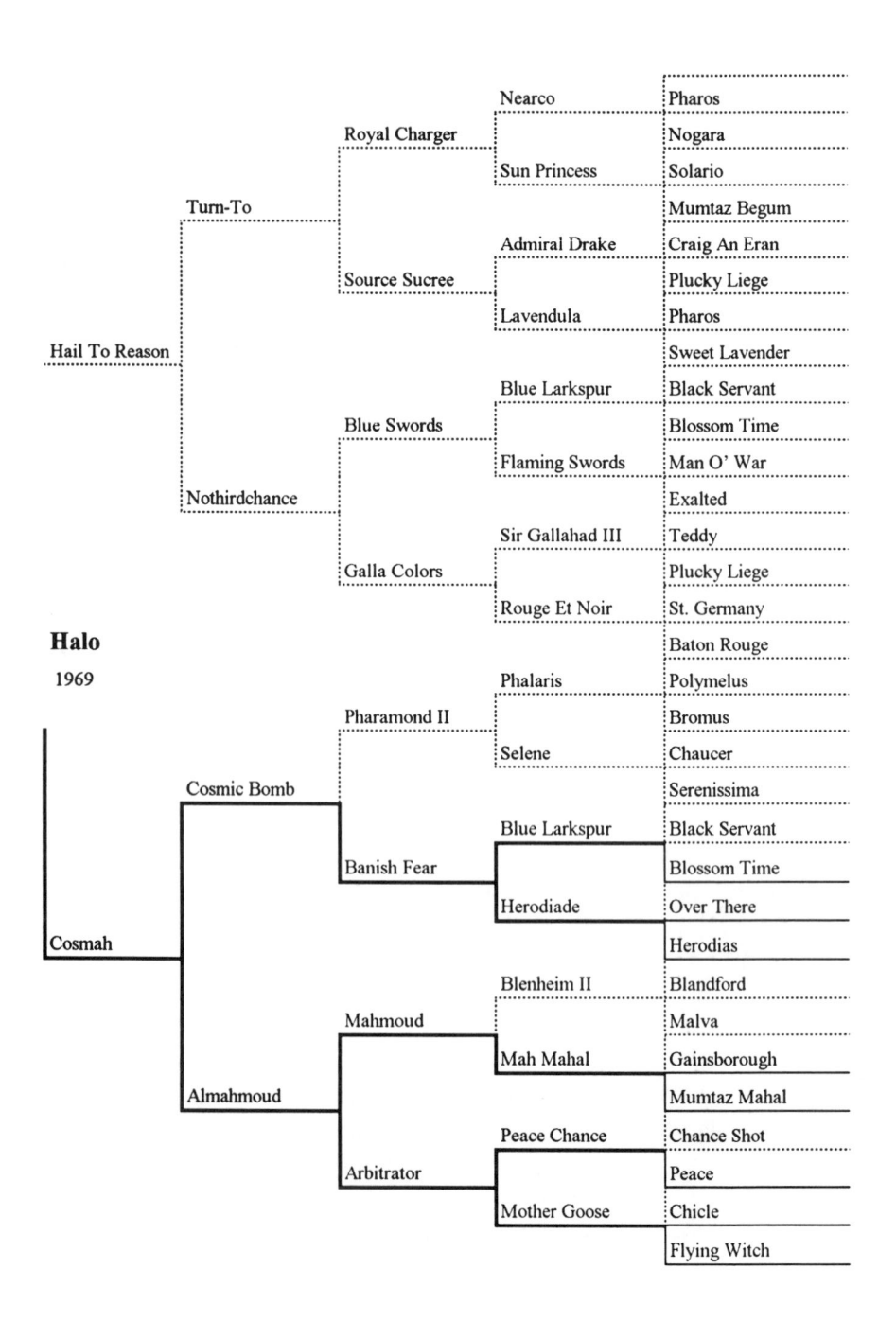

Hail To Reason	Turn-To	Royal Charger	Nearco	Pharos
				Nogara
			Sun Princess	Solario
				Mumtaz Begum
		Source Sucree	Admiral Drake	Craig An Eran
				Plucky Liege
			Lavendula	Pharos
				Sweet Lavender
	Nothirdchance	Blue Swords	Blue Larkspur	Black Servant
				Blossom Time
			Flaming Swords	Man O' War
				Exalted
		Galla Colors	Sir Gallahad III	Teddy
				Plucky Liege
			Rouge Et Noir	St. Germany
				Baton Rouge
Cosmah	Cosmic Bomb	Pharamond II	Phalaris	Polymelus
				Bromus
			Selene	Chaucer
				Serenissima
		Banish Fear	Blue Larkspur	Black Servant
				Blossom Time
			Herodiade	Over There
				Herodias
	Almahmoud	Mahmoud	Blenheim II	Blandford
				Malva
			Mah Mahal	Gainsborough
				Mumtaz Mahal
		Arbitrator	Peace Chance	Chance Shot
				Peace
			Mother Goose	Chicle
				Flying Witch

maternal granddam and grandsire, to paternal great-granddam and maternal great-granddam and great-grandsire.

The top line of the sire and the top line of the maternal grandsire are not relevant in this search as they are the Y chromosome lines.

For example, in Halo's pedigree (another outstanding large-hearted sire who has Mahmoud's heart going for him, with a dash of Blue Larkspur through his broodmare sire's dam, Banish Fear, a daughter of Blue Larkspur), the top side of his pedigree is not considered when looking for the large-heart he may pass on because it comes to him on the Y chromosome from his sire.

Even though it is on the Y chromosome line and the heart size cannot be passed this way, Halo's top side is a good example of large-hearted sires as well. His sire, Hail to Reason was a good broodmare sire, out of the dam, Nothirdchance, whose dam, Galla Colors, was a daughter of that outstanding broodmare sire, Sir Gallahad III, who went to Pocahontas through his dam, Plucky Liege. Hail to Reason's sire, Turn-To, also had large heart lines to Pocahontas through his dam, Source Sucree, a daughter of Admiral Drake, out of Plucky Liege, and on the tail-female line through the Swynford daughter, Sweet Lavender.

Halo's dam, Cosmah, has an outstanding large-heart pedigree. Her sire is Cosmic Bomb, who is out of Banish Fear, a daughter of Blue Larkspur, one of the four best large-heart lines, and she is out of Almahmoud, a daughter of another of the four, Mahmoud.

If a breeder were considering breeding to Halo, he would be an excellent choice. But to make sure that the genetic bases were covered, the breeder would need to bring a large-hearted mare to Halo with good heart lines to pass on if she produces a colt. This is where it is important to have measured that individual and to have carefully documented her pedigree and performance.

That way leaves as little as possible to chance.

Chapter 19

How to Measure Hearts

To find out what is inside a prospective athlete or breeding animal, you have to look. Science has given us ways to check the bones, joints, hearts, and lungs of potential athletes. Whether you use ultrasound or electrocardiograms, if you want to breed an outstanding performance athlete, or purchase a potential racehorse, you need to get all the available data about the engine that powers that horse.

A good healthy large heart in a racehorse is like having a high-powered V-8 engine in your car. You will never get left at the red light with a 351 Cleveland 4-bolt Main engine under your hood and a large heart in a racehorse means he will have a higher cardiac output and that means he will still have plenty of gas at the finish line.

Super horse Holy Bull, who was measured and found to have a large heart, tracing on his dam's side through Mahmoud, always amazed racegoers by his brilliant speed and seemingly effortless races. Following his win in the Blue Grass Stakes, he didn't even seem to be breathing hard after running away from the field.

When his trainer, Jimmy Croll, would work him in the morning, his speed always surprised because it seemed so effortless. It was hard to believe he was running as fast as he was when he didn't look as if he were putting out much effort at all.

Holy Bull had a very big and very effective engine powering him around the track. And he was generally carrying

Holy Bull
1991

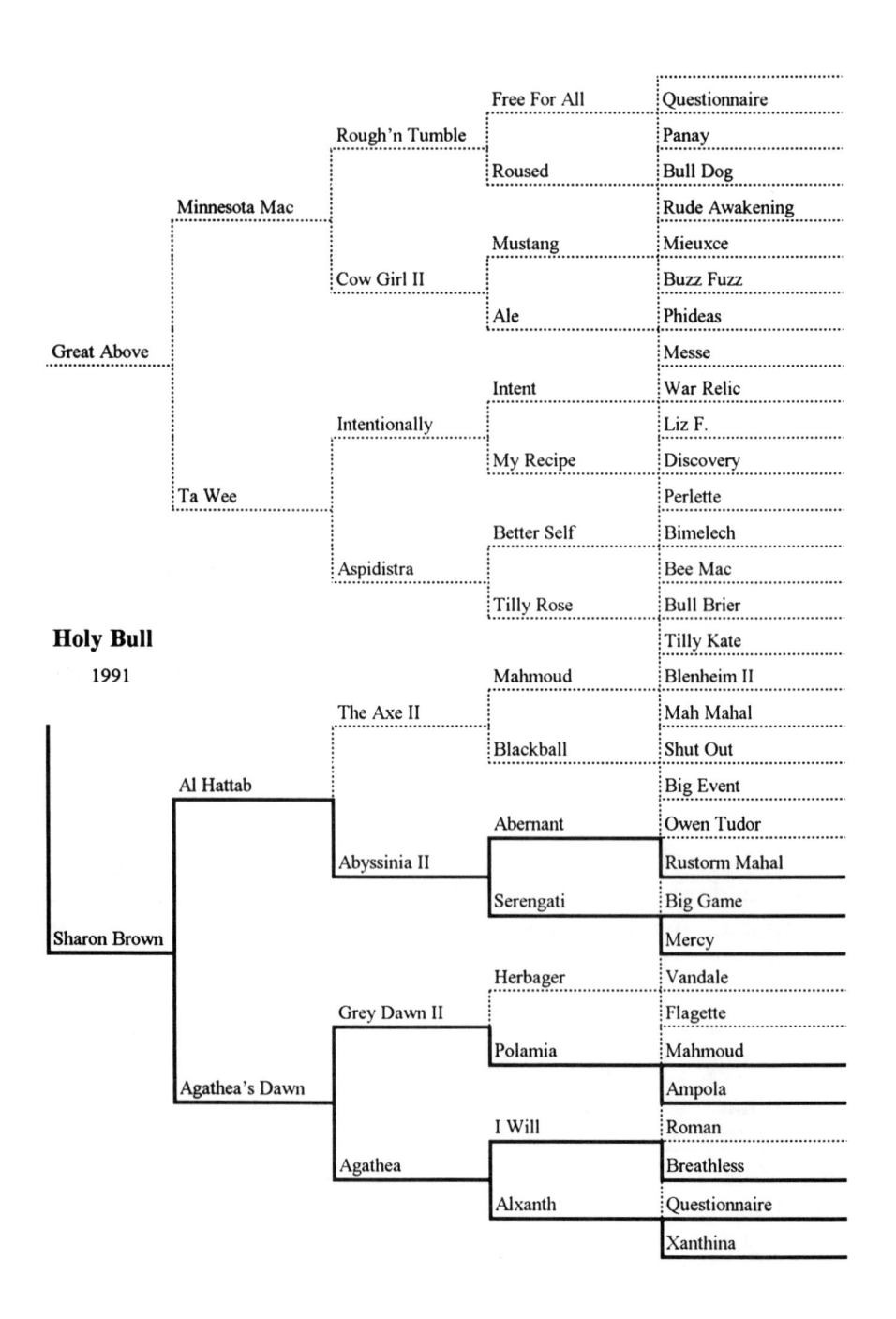

- Great Above
  - Minnesota Mac
    - Rough'n Tumble
      - Free For All
        - Questionnaire
        - Panay
      - Roused
        - Bull Dog
        - Rude Awakening
    - Cow Girl II
      - Mustang
        - Mieuxce
        - Buzz Fuzz
      - Ale
        - Phideas
        - Messe
  - Ta Wee
    - Intentionally
      - Intent
        - War Relic
        - Liz F.
      - My Recipe
        - Discovery
        - Perlette
    - Aspidistra
      - Better Self
        - Bimelech
        - Bee Mac
      - Tilly Rose
        - Bull Brier
        - Tilly Kate

- Sharon Brown
  - Al Hattab
    - The Axe II
      - Mahmoud
        - Blenheim II
        - Mah Mahal
      - Blackball
        - Shut Out
        - Big Event
    - Abyssinia II
      - Abernant
        - Owen Tudor
        - Rustorm Mahal
      - Serengati
        - Big Game
        - Mercy
  - Agathea's Dawn
    - Grey Dawn II
      - Herbager
        - Vandale
        - Flagette
      - Polamia
        - Mahmoud
        - Ampola
    - Agathea
      - I Will
        - Roman
        - Breathless
      - Alxanth
        - Questionnaire
        - Xanthina

150

an exercise rider that weighed around 150 pounds, a trick of Croll's to help condition him for whatever weight he had to carry. It will be interesting to see what his daughters can do.

Heart size and its importance in racing performance is still on the cutting edge in horse racing. It is a tool that has so far, only been used by the very wealthy - people like Robert Sangster, Earl Macke, and Pin Oak owner, Josephine Abercrombie.

It is something that is seen at the very top sales like Keeneland's July Select Sale and the Saratoga sale in August. The most common way of measuring the horses' hearts at the sales is by using an ultrasound machine in a manner developed by radiologist Norman Rantanen. Because the heart increases in size until the horse is four years old, the measuring of yearlings at the top sales is done with a mathematical formula to predict the final outcome. But when a yearling already has a large heart, the buyer knows he has a good one.

The genetic tracing project described in Part III of this book used the electrocardiogram so that it could compare its results with research already done by the Australians, who developed the use of the ECG in determining heart scores used in their research, and the work of the past 20 years using the ECG done by equine cardiologist, Dr. Frederick Fregin.

Using the electrocardiogram, Drs. James D. Steel and Anthony Stewart had found a linear correlation between the duration of the QRS complex (heart score) and the weight of the heart in studies conducted on Thoroughbreds and Standardbreds. Horses with high heart scores tended to race more successfully than horses with low heart scores in their studies. They demonstrated a similar relationship in humans in later studies.

In one of the measurements in the gene tracing project, a 14-month-old colt was measured to see the difference in size compared to the breeding and racing stock which were the major subjects of the study. He turned out to be one of those who had a large heart early in his development. At only 14 months, with more than two years left to grow, he already had a heart score of 130, which would be considered large in a fully-grown and trained racehorse.

Given the time left to grow and the research on size increases with age, this colt could very well develop into an adult with a heart score of at least 150, which would put him in very elite company. His pedigree line led to Citation, through his daughter, Beyond, on his dam's bottom line. His dam was a daughter of Prince John, who goes to Blue Larkspur, through his maternal granddam, Banish Fear, who is also found in Halo's pedigree.

It will be interesting to track this individual as he goes into training and see what happens to him. He is from Mountain Cat's first crop. His sire, Mountain Cat, who is out of a daughter of Key to the Mint, is also a large-hearted sire who is passing on his heart to his daughters. This colt is a good example of what can happen when you breed a mare with the right heart lines to a large-hearted sire.

While it is always best to select a mare for breeding with a good performance record, this isn't always necessary. There are always individuals, that for some reason - injury, finances, or whatever - didn't have outstanding performance records but still have outstanding pedigrees with the right heartlines.

An example is the mare Ride the Trails, by Prince John, who traces to Blue Larkspur through her paternal great-granddam, Banish Fear, and to Princequillo through her broodmare sire Sir Gaylord's dam, Somethingroyal, and to War Admiral, through her tail female line to her great-grandam, Portage, a daughter of War Admiral.

Ride the Trails never raced but she produced the champion, Cozzene, as well as black-type winning daughters, Mochila, Movin' Money, and Ivy Road, and winner Mesabi, all of whom have gone on to produce black-type winners.

Turf history is full of mares who either were never raced or who were unsuccessful at racing, but still went on to produce winners. Playmate, who only placed at four still produced the Irish champion two-year-old, Woodman, who has gone on to be a successful sire. Playmate carried the large-hearted X chromosome from her sire, Buckpasser out of Busanda, by War Admiral out of Businesslike, by Blue Larkspur. Buckpasser is one of the very best proponents of the large heart through his double copy dam.

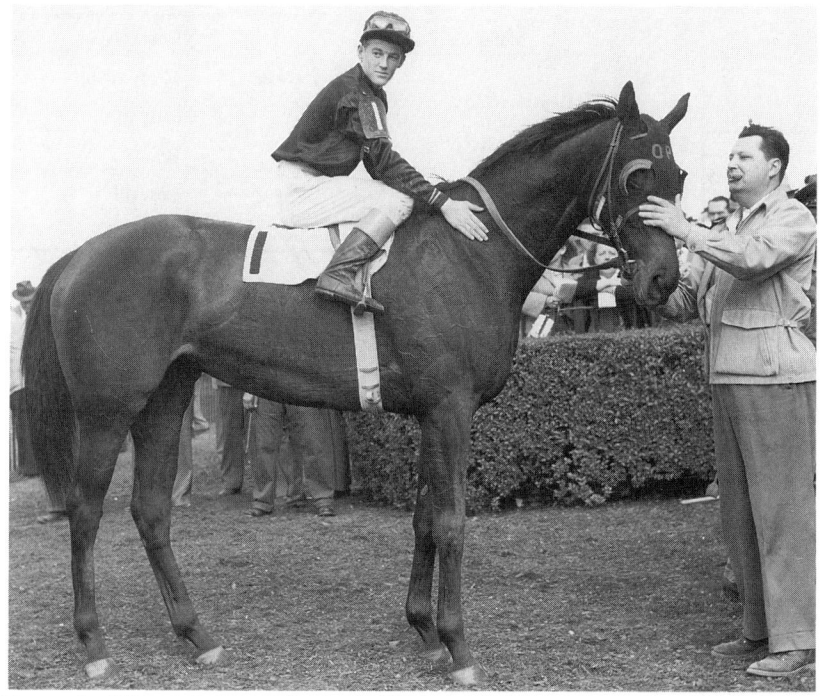

Busanda (War Admiral x Businesslike) the double copy dam of Buckpasser
Photo courtesy of the Keeneland Library

Using the ECG and autopsy reports, large hearts were found consistently in the maternal grandsons of Buckpasser.

Since 1953, electrocardiography has been used as a noninvasive technique to **determine the** heart size of racehorses. To do the procedure requires careful measurements of the QRS interval in each of the standard limb leads and calculation of the mean QRS duration in milliseconds, which is then referred to as the heart score.

In measurements of more than 120 horses, heart scores ranging from 103 (small) to 160 (very large) have been found.

Busanda
1947

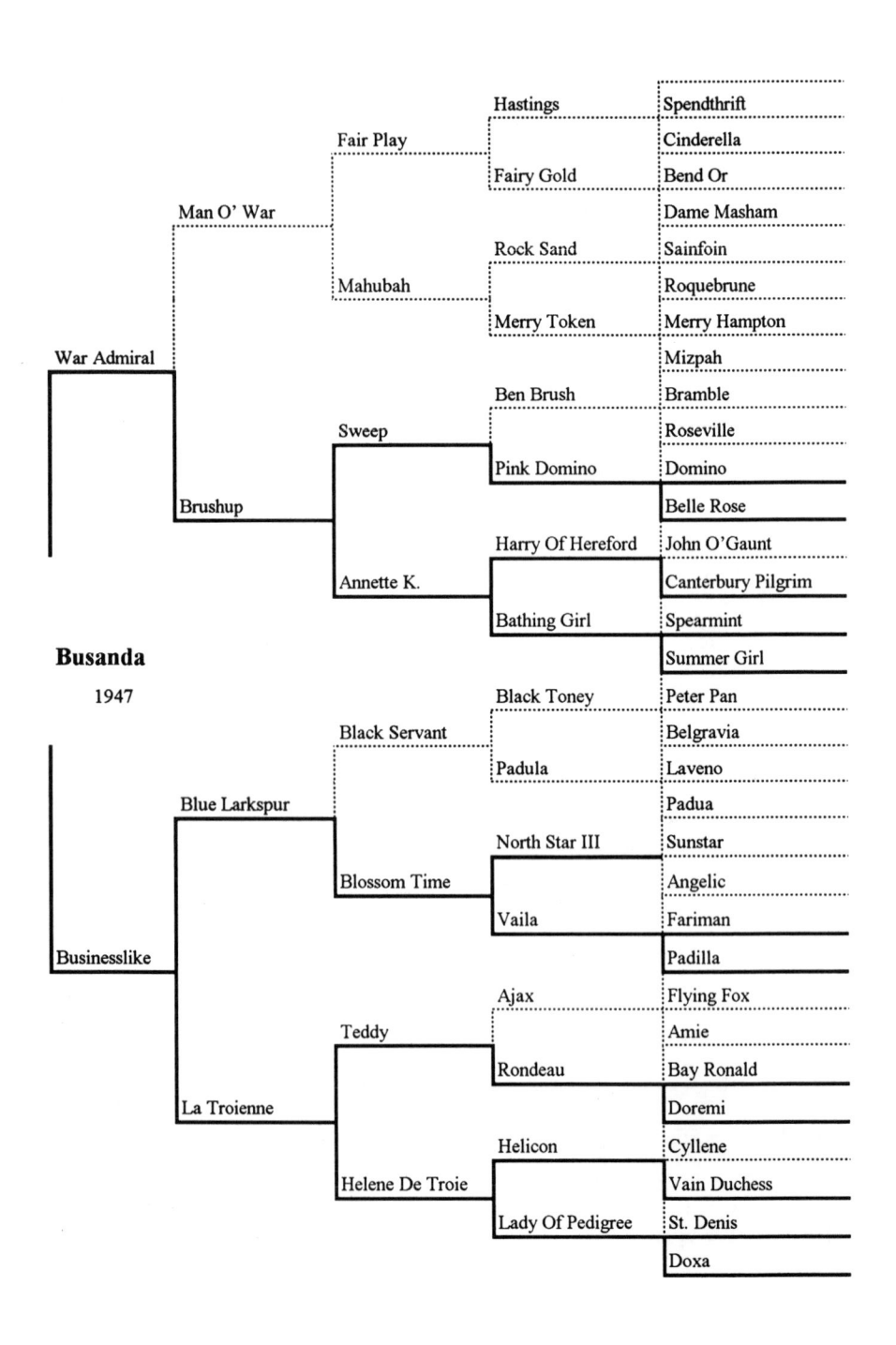

- War Admiral
  - Man O' War
    - Fair Play
      - Hastings
        - Spendthrift
        - Cinderella
      - Fairy Gold
        - Bend Or
        - Dame Masham
    - Mahubah
      - Rock Sand
        - Sainfoin
        - Roquebrune
      - Merry Token
        - Merry Hampton
        - Mizpah
  - Brushup
    - Sweep
      - Ben Brush
        - Bramble
        - Roseville
      - Pink Domino
        - Domino
        - Belle Rose
    - Annette K.
      - Harry Of Hereford
        - John O'Gaunt
        - Canterbury Pilgrim
      - Bathing Girl
        - Spearmint
        - Summer Girl

- Businesslike
  - Blue Larkspur
    - Black Servant
      - Black Toney
        - Peter Pan
        - Belgravia
      - Padula
        - Laveno
        - Padua
    - Blossom Time
      - North Star III
        - Sunstar
        - Angelic
      - Vaila
        - Fariman
        - Padilla
  - La Troienne
    - Teddy
      - Ajax
        - Flying Fox
        - Amie
      - Rondeau
        - Bay Ronald
        - Doremi
    - Helene De Troie
      - Helicon
        - Cyllene
        - Vain Duchess
      - Lady Of Pedigree
        - St. Denis
        - Doxa

In Stewart and Steel's studies, they reported individual heart scores from 86 to 146. Stewart said the largest heart score he has measured was 143.

While the gene tracing project has found larger heart scores than the Australians, it has had access to the very best bloodstock in the world. The horses with the very highest heart scores all track to the four largest heart lines, and were, unless stopped by injury, all top performers, including a number of champions.

In the 127 horses measured in the project, the heart score ranges broke down as follows:

Mares: Heart scores from 100 to 157 were recorded.

Stallions: Heart scores from 117 to 157 were recorded.

Two-year-olds in training: Heart scores from 117 to 133.

One yearling was measured at 14 months with a heart score of 130 and one three-year-old in training was measured carrying a heart score of 137.

There were 17 stallions measured; 10 two-year-olds in training; one yearling; one three-year-old in training; and 98 mares.

The smallest heart scores were found either in failed racehorses or in mares carrying a single copy. Two mares that were measured and found to have small-to-normal sized hearts had one X chromosome line with good heart lines and had produced large-hearted offspring. With single-copy mares, it simply depends on which X comes up as dominant in the genetic spin of the wheel.

In choosing an ECG to measure a horse's heart size, the heart score categories are: 103 and below are considered small; 104-to-117 are considered normal-sized; and, in fillies, 116 and up are considered large hearts, while colts are considered to have large hearts with heart scores from 120 and up.

"Electrocardiography, which once was the exclusive tool of the cardiologist, is a relatively inexpensive and noninvasive tool which can be used by the veterinary practitioner and his staff," said Dr. Frederick Fregin, who conducted all of the gene project measurements on the ECG.

"The form of the equine ECG will be altered significantly by variations in the activity of the autonomic nervous system (excitement for example) and by changes in forelimb positioning. It is important that the horse be examined in quiet, familiar surroundings, with the forelimbs kept parallel to each other and perpendicular to the long axis of the body."

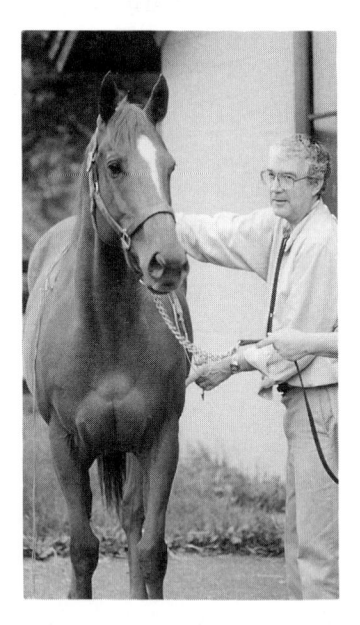

Dr. Fred Fregin, Director of the Marion duPont Scott Equine Medical Center measures the heart of Soviet Problem

Photo by Marianna Haun

In the study, most of the measurements were done in each horse's own stall, but some mares' were done in paddocks near their pasture. The most important thing was to keep them quiet in order to obtain a good tracing on the ECG. Nervous head-tossing or jerks or twitches could distort the tracing.

The author was involved in the study and her job was to be at the horse's head and keep him or her calm while Fregin listened for heart sounds and then set the ECG leads and ran the tape.

I must have a smell that horses relate to because they all liked to rest their noses on my chest, mares and stallions alike. When we were doing 53 horses in California in just a few days, the small of my back by the end of the day was killing me and the horse manager was worrying that my sweatshirt would act as a vector if any of the horses had any germs.

But it worked. Even Key to the Mint, who hadn't been in for a year and came in rearing, reacted positively to my smell and my voice with his eyes visibly softening and his lids drooping as he rested his nose on my chest. Gainesway's veterinarian, Norman Umphenour, said I was "mesmerizing" the stallion.

In describing the technique he uses with the ECG, Fregin said, "Patient cables with a total length of 20 to 25 feet are used to allow the ECG equipment to be placed in a remote location outside of the box stall. The limb and chest leads should be five feet in length and accommodate larger horses.

"Alligator clips fixed to the ECG leads may be attached directly to the skin after vigorous application of an electrode paste of gel. Discomfort to the horse will be minimized by smoothing (rounding off) the serrated edges of the alligator clips, by insuring that the maximum amount of skin is grasped, and by reducing tension or movement of the leads. The electrodes are placed on the caudal aspect of the forelimb approximately 15 cm below the level of the olecranon and on the hind limbs, distal or lateral to the stifle joint. The standard bipolar limb leads recorded are right foreleg and left foreleg (lead I), right foreleg and left hind leg (lead II), and left foreleg and left hind leg (lead III).

"The configuration of the wave forms in different leads depends on the direction and relative magnitude of the variations in the electrical forces generated during the cardiac cycle. These forces are determined primarily by the specialized conduction tissue (Purkinje fibers) and its influence on the spread of excitation through the myocardium. The wave forms are also influenced by the anatomic location and configuration of the heart, by the shape of the thorax, and by the electrical conductivity of the tissues between the heart and recording electrodes."

Norm Rantanen, one of the nation's top radiologists, who developed the use of two dimensional echocardiography (ultrasound) to measure the heart size of horses, said he has done comparison studies of the two methods, ECG and ultrasound, and found them consistent in their findings on heart size.

"We tried the technique that the Aussies use - the ECG which is what Fred (Fregin) is using," Rantanen said. "We also tried the ultrasound and they picked the top horses in any group that we did. (Dr.) Doug Byars did the ECGs. (Byars is director of the Internal Medicine Hospital of Hagyard-Davidson-McGee Equine Medicine and Surgery in Lexington, KY.) We did it on North Ridge yearlings. We went to Ireland and did a whole series of yearlings over there. Doug did the ECG and I did the ultrasound. He ranked his according to what he found and I ranked mine according to what I found. We always picked the top horses. The findings were very consistent."

Rantanen, who has measured nearly 4,000 horses since developing the use of ultrasound, said, "The best ones have the bigger hearts. That's what I've found over the years."

Rantanen started measuring hearts in the Lexington, Kentucky area in 1983.

"We used ultrasound," he said. "We knew we could do hearts. That was a no-brainer because they were doing it on people and if you can do it on people, you can do it on animals.

"When I first came to Lexington, I worked for two medical ultrasonographers. They had hired me to come to Lexington and develop the animal ultrasound. At that time, everybody was looking into exercise physiology and performance testing. It was the latest thing. We tried to promote that particular service and called in work daily from Washington state and a few other people and offered that to the owners and trainers and people in town as a way they could test their animals and learn something about their physiology. One of the things we were offering was cardiac tests.

"That's how I got started. That is when (veterinarian David) Lambert came to me. He asked me about the procedures I was doing and I told him. That's when he asked me if I would be interested in looking at some stock. We looked primarily at two-year-olds in training. I measured horses at Don and Linda Johnson's Crescent Farm. I scanned Night Shift, now standing in Europe. He was an unraced son of Northern Dancer and had a very large heart. He had surgery on his soft palate as a yearling that was screwed up and it ruined him for racing.

In developing his technique, Rantanen had the help of Dr. Anthony DeMaria, who was then the chief of cardiology at the University of Kentucky. "We had Tony out to help us with our technique," Rantanen said. "We hauled tapes to UK and Norton's Children's Hospital in Louisville where they allowed us to use their measuring devices. With their help, I came up with a technique that was reproducible in the same horse at different times and also between horses because I knew exactly where to go inside the heart."

Rantanen was not surprised at the consistency of heart size found in hearts on certain lines in our project.

"I knew that because of the information the Australians had published," he said. "And I believe that the broodmare has a lot to do with it. I knew there was something there, but I just didn't have the wherewithal to follow it up. I didn't have the opportunity to follow a lot of family lines. I didn't have the budget to do that.

"We did a lot at North Ridge Farm for Franklin Groves. We went there and did his yearling crops. We ranked them from top to bottom. We were hoping that he would use that to dictate which horses that he sold, but he didn't do that. A lot of horses ended up being sold to people that were right at the top of the list we made.

"When horses have very large hearts, you can see them as yearlings. Yearlings are identifiable."

Rantanen said when he started looking at horses' hearts, it was primarily for people who were looking for horses to race. "We looked at two-year-olds in training," he said. "After that, we started looking at younger horses. I also looked at some broodmares for Robert Sangster.

"But it was really hard to get people to fund it. I did a lot of stuff for nothing. I worked my butt off for months and months and months with no funding just to get the technique down."

Today, Rantanen credits Lambert with having the best technique for measuring hearts. "He took the technique I developed and was able to get the financial backing to do the statistical work on it," Rantanen said. "So he knows the most. But he is doing it as a private venture and he is certainly not going to divulge his techniques."

In a report validating the use of two-dimensional echocardiography of the horse as used by Rantanen, K. Voros, J.R. Holmes, and Christine Gibbs from the University of Bristol in Bristol, England, wrote in the Equine Veterinary Journal that during ultrasound examinations, the transducer is placed between the ribs either on the right or left side of the chest where bone and overlying lung interference can be avoided.

"The 4th and 5th intercostal spaces are referred to as caudal and the 3rd as cranial transducer locations," the report said. "In the latter position it is helpful to draw the relevant foreleg forward.

"To permit production of repeatable images of the same tomographic planes, intracardiac reference points were established. Current nomenclature in two-dimensional echocardiographic examinations refers to a long axis and a short axis view. These are really longitudinal and transverse planes respectively. The right and left long axis view were obtained with the scan plane orientated parallel to the longitudinal cardiac axis, and the short axis views were achieved by directing the beam plane perpendicular to the longitudinal cardiac axis.

"By moving the transducer from the apex to the base, several distinct short axis levels of the heart can be imaged and are classified according to relevant anatomical landmarks. From below upwards, they are referred to as papillary muscle, chordae tendineae, mitral valve, and aortic levels respectively. In all views caudo-medial or cranio-medial angulation of the

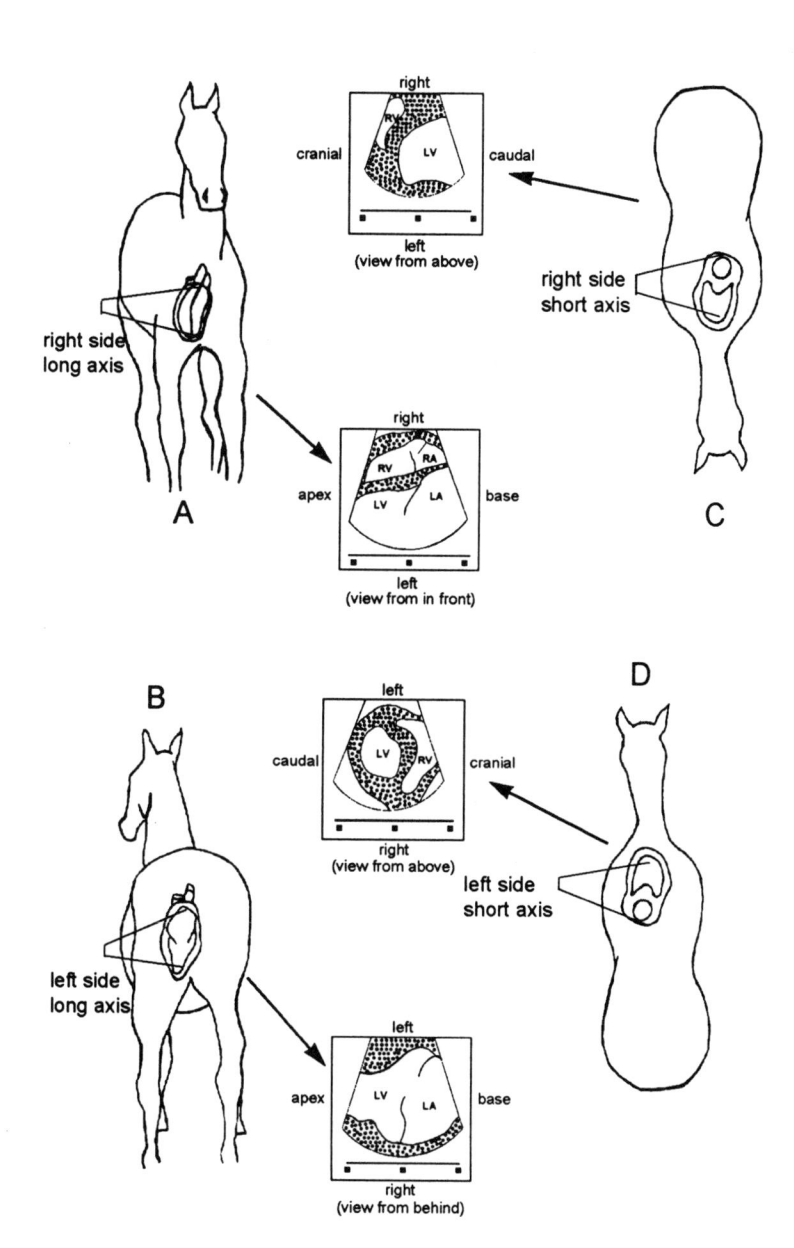

A) Schematic illustration of imaging and projection of long axis planes recorded from the right side of the chest. The scan is viewed from in front of the horse. RA: right atrium; RV: right ventricle; LA: left atrium; LV: left ventricle. B) Schematic illustration of imaging and projection of long axis planes recorded from the left side of the chest. The scan is viewed from behind the horse. LA: left atrium; LV: left ventricle. C) Schematic illustration of imaging and projections of short axis planes recorded from the right side of the chest. The scan is viewed from above the horse. RV: right ventricle; LV: left ventricle. D) Schematic illustration of imaging and projections of short axis planes recorded from the left side of the chest. The scan is viewed from above the horse. RV: right ventricle; LV: left ventricle.

beam plane may be necessary to examine the whole range of cardiac structure.

"Regardless of which side of the chest the transducer was placed, the images were displayed on the video screen with the apex of the heart always to the left and the base (atria, great vessels) to the right. Because of this orientation, long axis images taken from the right side of the chest were projected as through the encountered tomographic planes were viewed from the cranial to the caudal part of the heart and images obtained from the left side were viewed from the caudal to the cranial part of the heart.

"Short axis images recorded from either the right or the left side of the chest were projected as though the encountered tomographic planes were viewed from above, namely from the base to the apex of the heart. Thus, short axis images obtained from the right side of the chest were displayed on the video screen with cranial echoes to the left and with cranial echoes to the right side of the screen and those taken from the left side with cranial echoes to the right and caudal echoes to the left of the screen."

The study demonstrated that two-dimensional echocardiogry (ultrasound) was an accurate anatomical evaluation of the equine heart.

The use of the ultrasound is one more way of measuring a potential athlete's heart. Gaining that valuable information, which when coupled with a pedigree predicting good heart line inheritability, can add that much more of an edge for success in the very expensive and competitive world of racing.

Chapter 20

Current Research

Following the discovery of Secretariat's heart and the beginning of the research on the X-Factor and heart size in Thoroughbred racehorses and bloodstock, Dr. Thomas Swerczek, head pathologist at the University of Kentucky, began compiling data on heart size at autopsy.

When Easy Goer died, Swerczek did his autopsy and found a large heart. Easy Goer, who was out of a Buckpasser daughter, did not have a heart as large as Secretariat's or Sham's, but he had a very large heart.

"It weighed between 15 and 16 pounds," Swerczek said, making the heart near twice the normal size of 8 1/2 pounds.

Swerczek also did the autopsy on the champion mare, Althea, a daughter of Alydar, out of Courtly Dee, whose dam was a daughter of War Admiral.

"Althea's heart looked very much like a stallion's heart," Swerczek said. "It was a very big heart, comparable to the size of Easy Goer's heart."

In inheriting her large heart, Althea had a choice of one of two X chromosomes from her dam, Courtly Dee, and one from her sire, Alydar, who carried the Blue Larkspur heartline.

On her dam's side, the large-hearted X chromosome would come from either Never Bend, Courtly Dee's sire, who also carried the Blue Larkspur heartline through his maternal great-granddam, Bloodroot, a daughter of Blue Larkspur, or the one from her dam, Tulle, a daughter of War Admiral, out of the double copy mare, Judy-Rae, by *Beau Pere out of the *Sir

Gallahad III daughter, Betty Derr. In Courtly Dee's pedigree, all lines led to Pocahontas.

That means that Althea had two shots at the Blue Larkspur heart and one shot at the War Admiral heart in the genetic spin of the wheel at the moment of her creation.

Given the similarity in heart size that she shared with Easy Goer, that might mean that she carried the War Admiral. But it isn't certain.

In the study, it was found that War Admiral and Blue Larkspur hearts were of similar large sizes. There was much inbreeding of these two heart lines, especially through Buckpasser, whose dam, Busanda was a daughter of War Admiral out of a daughter of Blue Larkspur.

In addition to collecting autopsy data, the process has begun at the University of Kentucky to look for the genetic marker for this trait. Funding for the search is yet to be secured.

In preparation for that work, though, blood was collected from all of the horses measured and preliminary blood work has been completed, separating the DNA from each sample and storing it for the next step.

According to UK geneticist Gus Cothran, the genetic marker search will follow the same protocal the university uses in searching for specific disease characteristics.

"Basically, it is called bulk segregant analysis," Cothran said. "You take DNA samples from horses that do not have the trait of interest and mix them all together. Then you take DNA samples from horses that have the trait of interest and mix them together. Then you test them for a series of genetic markers-ones that are easy to find. For related individuals with different heart sizes, you pool the samples to mask the individual variability, then any difference you find between the two pools has a very high probability of being related to the trait.

"What you are hoping to see is a positive product in one group and no product or negative result in the other. It doesn't matter which one because once you find that, then you do what we call cloning and trying to find out exactly what the gene is. Once you find a difference that is consistently showing up where the group that has the trait shows one pattern and the group that doesn't show the trait shows the other pattern, then you can be comfortable that the marker you have found is in fact associated with that characteristic.

"It might not actually be the gene itself, but it should be close enough that it should give you a place that you could really start looking for it," he said.

"There is no way to predict how long this would take. Eventually, you are almost certain to find something, but you might have to do 1,000 tests to find it. Or, you might get it on the first try. The main cost of finding it is paying someone to do the tests."

The search will also involve even more in-depth pedigree research and analysis.

"You have to know what the progeny has done," Cothran said. "That is why a marker can be so valuable. You don't have to wait for all these progeny results to know what you've got.

"With double copy mares (homozygous), you have the highest mathematical probability that they will pass on the characteristic to all of their progeny.

"There are good Blue Hen mares here that have one or more links and you look at their progeny and some are good and some are bad. If this characteristic is working the way it seems to be working, that means that some of these mares are heterozygous (single copy).

"That means they may or may not express the large heart, but they only carry the characteristic on one X chromosome. This means that only 50 percent of their offspring, by chance, would have the large heart. It would depend upon which X chromosome they give their progeny. In the case of a filly, if they got the small heart X from their dam and the large-heart X from their sire, it would depend upon which X chromosome was dominant as to whether she would express the large-hearted characteristic. But even if she didn't express the large heart, she would be a 'carrier,' capable of passing it on to one-half of her progeny."

In addition to tracking the large heart through pedigrees, demonstrating strong evidence of sex linkage, and identifying the four largest heart lines, the study has also opened up other possible research areas, particularly in the way that physical characteristics seem to follow the heart size down the X chromosome.

Given the genetic discovery at Cornell University demonstrating that the Y chromosome has more influence on the uterine environment and the X chromosome has more influence in the formation of the body of the horse, this could be a major area of research leading to important discoveries impacting on the study of heart conditions in humans.

Chapter 21

Cher Chez la Femme

In summing up what was learned in this project, the importance of looking at the bottom of the pedigree cannot be stressed enough.

Given what has been learned about inherited characteristics on the X chromosome, it is time to put centuries of sexism in terms of Thoroughbred pedigrees behind us. The dam is every bit as important, if not more so, than the sire. With the heart, possible physical characteristics, and a pattern of performance traveling down the X chromosome trail, all X lines in both the sire and the dam must be taken into account.

Because breeders have long known the importance of a good broodmare sire, the large heart has been able to make its way down through generations of outstanding racehorses. But with newly gained knowledge about the X chromosome, it can now be seen that when it comes to raising sons of champions, the mare must bring the large heart into the mix.

Given the possible choices on the X-chromosome lines, it is important to cover all the bases. That means not only a good broodmare sire, but a good heartline on the tail-female line and through the sire of the maternal granddam.

When breeding fillies, it is also important to make sure that the sire has a large heart.

Hopefully, what has been learned will put to rest the practice of condemning a sire that doesn't reproduce himself in his sons, but does give great heart to his daughters.

Sires like Citation, Omaha, and Whirlaway would have benefited from the knowledge we have today of where their great hearts came from. If they had been mated to large hearted double copy mares, their sons might have equalled or surpassed their daughters, and come closer to equalling their sire's outstanding racing feats.

Secretariat, because of his enormous heart, has finally made the world listen. When bred to large-hearted mares, he produced sons like Pancho Villa, General Assembly, Risen Star, and Medaille D'Or.

But his mighty heart was reserved for his daughters, who in turn passed it on to maternal grandsons like A.P. Indy, Summer Squall, Storm Cat, Dehere, and Gone West, to name just a few.

A broodmare sire is one because he passes on his best traits through his daughters. That is to say he passes on his traits on the X chromosome. Given the small size of the Y chromosome, it is not surprising that there is very little passed on it as compared to the much larger X chromosome.

Given a mare's two X chromosomes, it is easy to see why a mare carrying the large heart on both X chromosomes is worth her weight in gold. As long as she is bred to an outstanding stallion with a large heart, she will always produce a winner.

Given what we have found in terms of the large heart passing from the sire to his daughter, the 1996 Hambletonian takes on new meaning. In that race, two of the outstanding Standardbred sire, Valley Victory's progeny, a son, Lindy Lane, and a daughter, Continentalvictory, battled for the win. Continentalvictory, who had tied the world record in her preliminary heat earlier in the day, had enough heart left to beat her sire's son to the finish line.

Epilogue

The Secretariat Story

Secretariat, who gave new meaning to the term "great heart," was a physically beautiful horse.

When owner, Helen "Penny" Chenery, first saw him when he was 10 days old, she immediately thought, "Show horse, not race horse."

Explaining her first impression of the colt, Chenery said, "He looked like a Quarter horse baby. We were used to a rangier type, nothing so rounded and fully-packed. He was certainly the body type we hoped to get. But anything that had three white stockings and a bright chestnut coat and a perfectly straight nose, you just think, 'Oh, that belongs in the show ring,'"

As a yearling in the pasture with the other colts, Secretariat dominated the field.

"When he was turned out," Chenery said, "he was the star of the lot. He was the leader. I believe that the foal inherits the dam's herd position. Secretariat was out of a dominant mare, so he would be dominant."

Secretariat was foaled on March 30, 1970, at The Meadow in Virginia, where his dam, Somethingroyal had been raised. Chenery said she didn't remember much about Somethingroyal as a young horse because she was busy at the time raising her own babies.

"I did know that she was wonderful looking," Chenery said. "I did know enough to know that Princequillos were wonderful looking horses. Somethingroyal always had great-looking foals. My father bought her dam, Imperatrice, in Maryland. She was already a stakes winner who had produced a stakes winner when Dad bought her. She, too, was a great-looking horse and she lived to be 32.

"We had some nice broodmares. With us, it wasn't a case where one or two mares were going to carry the farm. When Secretariat was foaled, we had Iberia, who was Riva Ridge's dam; Syrian Sea, who was Secretariat's full sister, who was by then a producer, and Gay Matelda, also."

The Meadow raised two Kentucky Derby winners in a row. Riva Ridge, who won the Derby in 1972, was foaled by Iberia when she was 17. Somethingroyal was 18 when she had Secretariat, who won the Derby in 1973.

When Secretariat went to the training center as a yearling in August of 1971, Lucien Laurin had just been training for Meadow Stable for a couple of months.

"We start to break them in September," Chenery said. "We go with them through Thanksgiving, and if the weather is good, up to Christmas. When it was time to turn them out, Lucien came down and brought our vet because Secretariat had a tiny splint. Secretariat always had good legs, with no problems, but he really did have a tiny splint then and Lucien said he wanted to take him down to Florida.

"He said, 'I want to take this one to stay with me'. Otherwise, he would have been turned out for the winter. That was the right decision because he was going to be a big horse. And Lucien knew Sir Gaylord (Secretariat's half-brother) and he would have put on too much weight to take back off if he had been turned out.

"Lucien had only trained for me from June of that year and we had more than one trainer at the same time. He may have thought, 'I just better take that Bold Ruler colt with me.' Also, Secretariat had a curious mind and it was really much better for him to stay occupied."

Chenery's father, Christopher Chenery, a financier who had made his fortune running utilities companies, became ill with Alzheimer's and Penny began running the farm in 1967. Her father entered the hospital in 1968 and he never left. He would die in early January 1973, before Secretariat won the Kentucky Derby.

"I didn't get married early and my father was disappointed," Penny said. "After a while, he said, 'You have no marketable skills and you are not married.' So, he sent me to Columbia Graduate School of Business. He said, 'You will one day inherit money. You should learn how to manage it.'

"When the time came, I did know the basic elements of running a business. I could read a balance sheet. I could understand the accounting. I could read a contract and that was all because my father had foresight.

"I think he knew that my brother was never going to run the farm. He was an economist and just not bit interested. My sister was involved in real estate. Of course, by the time my moment came, she was available, but it was too late to change his plan."

When Chenery began running the farm for her father, it was considered unusual for a woman to run a Thoroughbred operation.

"There were lots of woman owners," she said, "but usually their names were on the horses' papers, and their husbands ran the business. When I started running the farm, I was still living in Colorado, raising my family, so I had to run it from a long distance."

In 1973, after her father's death in January, the issue of estate taxes became a concern and it was decided to syndicate Secretariat.

"When we syndicated him, I wanted to make it a flat $200,000 a share. But Claiborne didn't want it that much more than Buckpasser. He had been $180,000 a share. Secretariat's price of $190,000 per share was the highest of any syndication up to that time."

"Poor Seth. He had just taken the reins of Claiborne. He was 23 years old," Chenery said, "and had been handed this really daunting task and the first few people he called turned him down. But he was the hero of that deal. He got the job done.

Seth's father, A.B. 'Bull' Hancock, had died in the fall of 1972, naming Seth as president of Claiborne.

"Afterwards, people would say to me, 'But you didn't ask so and so,' and I would say, 'I didn't do that (contact investors). That was not my job. Of course, Seth turned to the clients of Claiborne. One of the people left out was Joan Payson. She didn't get a share, so her cousin, Alfred Vanderbilt, sold her half a share because he thought it was so wrong that she not be included.

"If I had more experience in syndicating a stallion, I would have given more thought to the important players in the business. But Seth and I were both brand new at this. Seth's list had the Claiborne patrons. I included some of my personal friends like Laddie Dance and his wife. Another couple that trained with Lucien had a share.

"Anybody in the horse business or breeding business could see how new I was to this. There is so much to learn if you don't know the horse business. And I obviously didn't know the business. It meant a lot to me not to foul up.

"Today I could do it better and so could Seth."

In campaigning Secretariat, one of Chenery's favorite races was the Bay Shore Stakes, his first race as a three-year-old.

"I loved the Bay Shore," Chenery said. "He had gone to Florida for the winter and shipped north for the race and it was lousy weather. We didn't know what he would be like as a three-year-old. He had gotten much bolder. In the race, he had to come, not from very far out of it, but far enough that he had to get around two horses and they were in his way. So he just split horses. He streaked between them and won by 4 1/2 lengths."

While being impressed by his race, Chenery was concerned about the way he ran between those two horses.

"He had been set down in the Champagne (Stakes) for bothering Stop the Music and I had really pouted a lot about that. So I was sure the stewards were going to do something about the way he split those two horses. But they didn't."

Secretariat went on to have an amazing three-year-old season, winning the Triple Crown, setting a world record in the

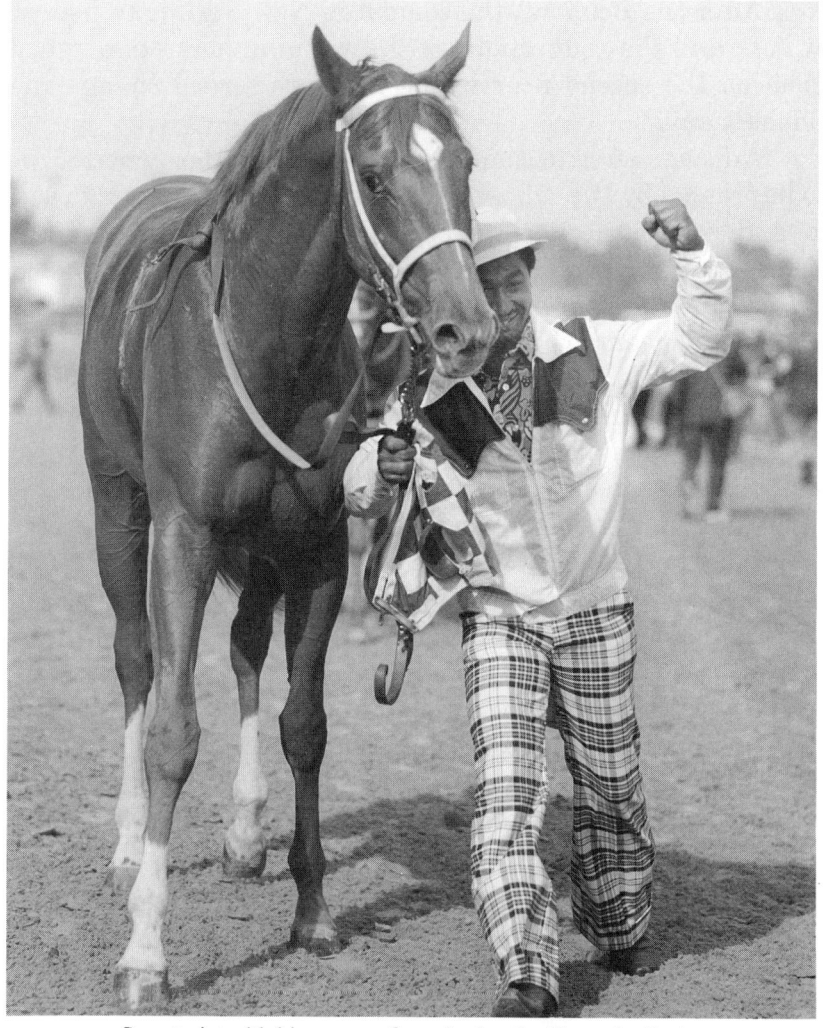

Secretariat with his groom after winning the Kentucky Derby
Photo courtesy of Penny Chenery

Marlboro Cup, winning the Man O' War Stakes on turf in course-record time, and ending his career in Canada with a 6-1/2 length victory in the Canadian International Championship.

The highlight of Secretariat's racing career, winning the first Triple Crown in 25 years, produced the crowning moment for Chenery as well.

"After the Belmont, the custom in New York is to take the owners and the connections of the winning horse to a private room on the second floor where they are served champagne," Chenery said.

"Anyone is free to come and congratulate the owners. I was so impressed by the caliber of people who took the time to come in and congratulate me. People like Jock Whitney and his sister, Joan Payson of Greentree Stud, and Paul Mellon. That did as much for me as anything in Secretariat's career. That was the moment of recognition that he wasn't just another Bold Ruler. The fact was that we had taken a Bold Ruler and set a track record at a mile and a half. Everybody had said Bold Rulers wouldn't go that far. And it wasn't just that we got lucky. We had really done something. And the true horsemen came to tell me so. It was just wonderful."

Of course, Chenery said, there were also a number of "very relieved" shareholders. "They had gotten their money's worth."

Chenery said she didn't think of Secretariat's victory in the Triple Crown in terms of herself.

"I was there because I was managing Dad's horse. I knew that I had failed to 'mess up,' " she said with a laugh.

The true magnitude of the fame Secretariat would achieve in his lifetime and even after death is still unfolding for Chenery.

"It is still developing in my mind the extent of what this horse means to people. It was not only the track records. It seems that everybody will come and tell me that they saw him or that they cried at the Belmont or that they were at the Derby. They don't want anything from me. They want me to hear their memories. It's like one of those moments in time frozen in people's memories.

"He really became almost a cult figure after he retired to stud. I think a lot of it was because Claiborne was so gracious about letting people go see him. I give them a lot of credit. It didn't increase their business, but they understood their obligation as a conservator of a racing legend.

"He got enormous fan mail. I still get letters and people will send me things for sign. I still get pictures."

In spite of his racing success, Secretariat suffered some defeats, too. After winning a specially written race, the Arlington Invitational Stakes, on June 30, just 21 days after winning the Triple Crown at Belmont Park, Secretariat finished second to Onion in the Whitney Stakes at Saratoga, known in racing circles as the "graveyard of favorites."

Allen Jerkens, trainer of Onion, would upset Secretariat a second time with Prove Out on a sloppy track in the Woodward Stakes, that year.

Secretariat didn't like to lose.

"If he didn't win a race, he would go back to the barn, put his head in the corner and refuse to come to the webbing," Chenery said. "He would be mad at himself. 'Did that wrong.' I think they know when they get beat. I think they know when the rider stands up and they're not in the lead, that they haven't done it right."

But despite those setbacks, Secretariat mainly did it right.

After appearing on the cover of three national magazines - Sports Illustrated, Newsweek, and Time - the public was clamoring to see more of the "Big Red." In another specially written race, designed specifically for television, Secretariat delivered in a big way.

The race was originally conceived as a exhibition between two Kentucky Derby winners - Secretariat and his stablemate, Riva Ridge. But it was then opened up as an invitational. Seven horses competed, including Key to the Mint, Onion, and *Cougar II.

But it was Secretariat's show all the way. He hooked Riva Ridge in the stretch and ran away from the field to a 3 1/2-length victory, setting a world record of 1:45 2/5 for nine furlongs on the dirt.

In his final two starts, Secretariat competed on grass. Talking about that time, Chenery said, "He had already won the Triple Crown and then we had the disaster of the summer at Saratoga where he had been beaten. Following that, he was rested briefly. Then there was the excitement of bringing him back to racing form to run in the Marlboro Cup where he set a world record. After that, what was there left to do?

"So we worked him on the grass and he worked fine. His second to last start was in the Man O' War Stakes at Belmont Park. I had gone to the Arc, returning the day of the race. I got off the plane and went right to Belmont Park.

"He not only triumphed on the grass, but he romped home. He just loved it. He was so happy. He set a track record of 2:24.4 (for 1 1/2 miles on turf) which still stands. He just added a new dimension.

"We were getting so close to when we were going to have to retire him. I cherish that race because it was almost the last run and we found out more about him.

"Then, of course, he went to Canada. It was so bittersweet because we knew it was his last race. The weather turned and you could hardly see him. He was silhouetted against the light when he crossed the finish line.

"Ronnie didn't ride him because he'd been set down. Eddie Maple rode and he was scared to death that he would blow the last race. He was just ashen. No smile. Eddie's kind of laconic anyway, but generally, there is a twinkle. But you could not get a laugh out of Eddie that day until it was all over.

"And, bless his heart, it was lousy racing condition and there was pressure to have a track record." Secretariat won the race in the rain by 6 1/2 lengths, just one second slower than the course record.

"Once again, I was proud of him. But there it was. That was it. It was all over."

But it wasn't over.

The Big Red Machine's finest contribution to his racing community was yet to come. More than any other factor, his autopsy would trigger the search for the X-factor.

Appendix

To aid readers in researching their own horses' pedigrees, we have enclosed a number of five-cross pedigrees of some of the most outstanding Thoroughbred lines. Because of space considerations, not every large-hearted line is enclosed, but there should be enough variety to give the breeder or racehorse owner a good jumping off spot to research his or her own horse's heart line.

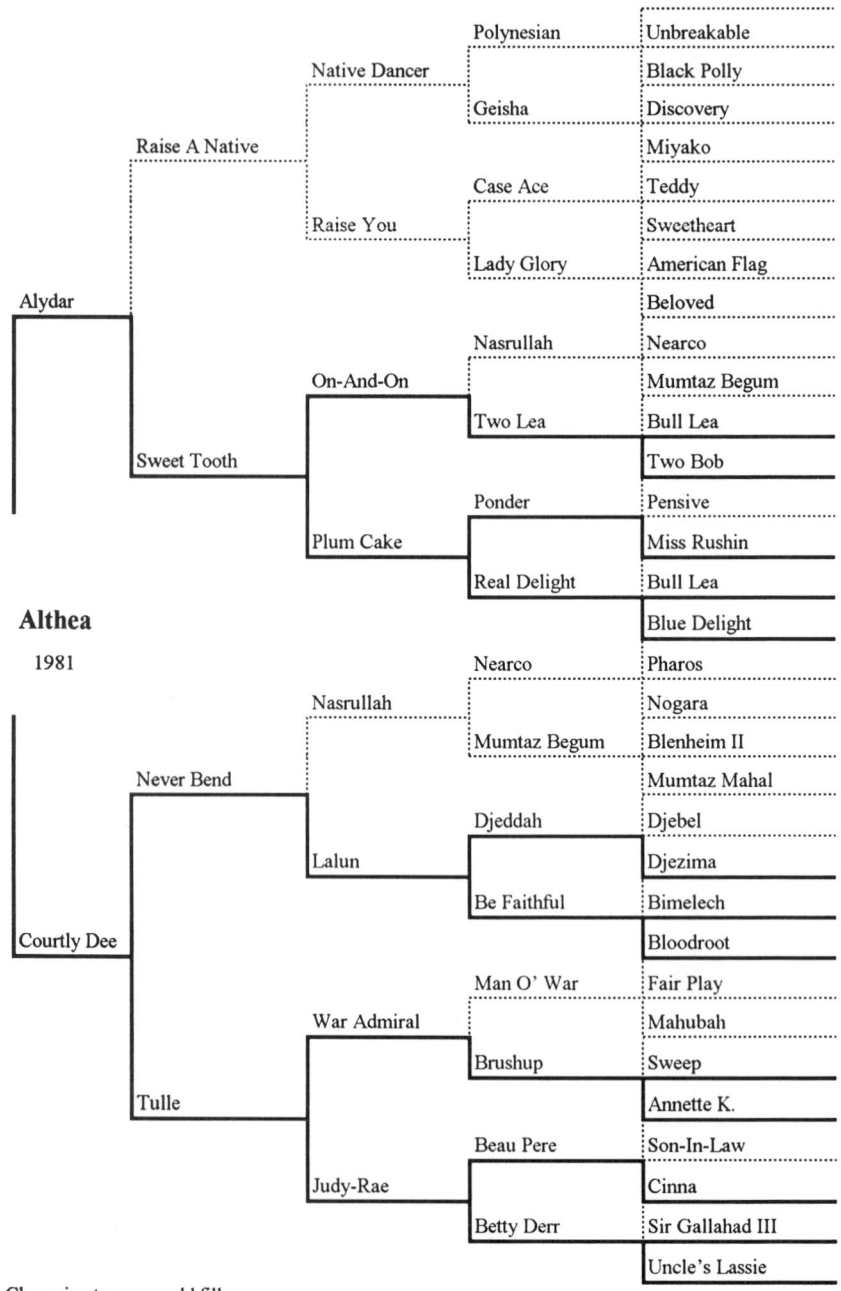

```
                                            ┌─ Polynesian ──┬─ Unbreakable
                          ┌─ Native Dancer ─┤               └─ Black Polly
                          │                 └─ Geisha ──────┬─ Discovery
        ┌─ Raise A Native ┤                                 └─ Miyako
        │                 │                 ┌─ Case Ace ────┬─ Teddy
        │                 └─ Raise You ─────┤               └─ Sweetheart
        │                                   └─ Lady Glory ──┬─ American Flag
─ Alydar ┤                                                  └─ Beloved
        │                                   ┌─ Nasrullah ───┬─ Nearco
        │                 ┌─ On-And-On ─────┤               └─ Mumtaz Begum
        │                 │                 └─ Two Lea ─────┬─ Bull Lea
        └─ Sweet Tooth ───┤                                 └─ Two Bob
                          │                 ┌─ Ponder ──────┬─ Pensive
                          └─ Plum Cake ─────┤               └─ Miss Rushin
                                            └─ Real Delight ┬─ Bull Lea
                                                            └─ Blue Delight
```

Althea
1981

```
                                            ┌─ Nearco ──────┬─ Pharos
                          ┌─ Nasrullah ─────┤               └─ Nogara
                          │                 └─ Mumtaz Begum ┬─ Blenheim II
        ┌─ Never Bend ────┤                                 └─ Mumtaz Mahal
        │                 │                 ┌─ Djeddah ─────┬─ Djebel
        │                 └─ Lalun ─────────┤               └─ Djezima
        │                                   └─ Be Faithful ─┬─ Bimelech
─ Courtly Dee ┤                                             └─ Bloodroot
        │                                   ┌─ Man O' War ──┬─ Fair Play
        │                 ┌─ War Admiral ───┤               └─ Mahubah
        │                 │                 └─ Brushup ─────┬─ Sweep
        └─ Tulle ─────────┤                                 └─ Annette K.
                          │                 ┌─ Beau Pere ───┬─ Son-In-Law
                          └─ Judy-Rae ──────┤               └─ Cinna
                                            └─ Betty Derr ──┬─ Sir Gallahad III
                                                            └─ Uncle's Lassie
```

Champion two-year-old filly
Earned $1,275,255

Alydar
1975

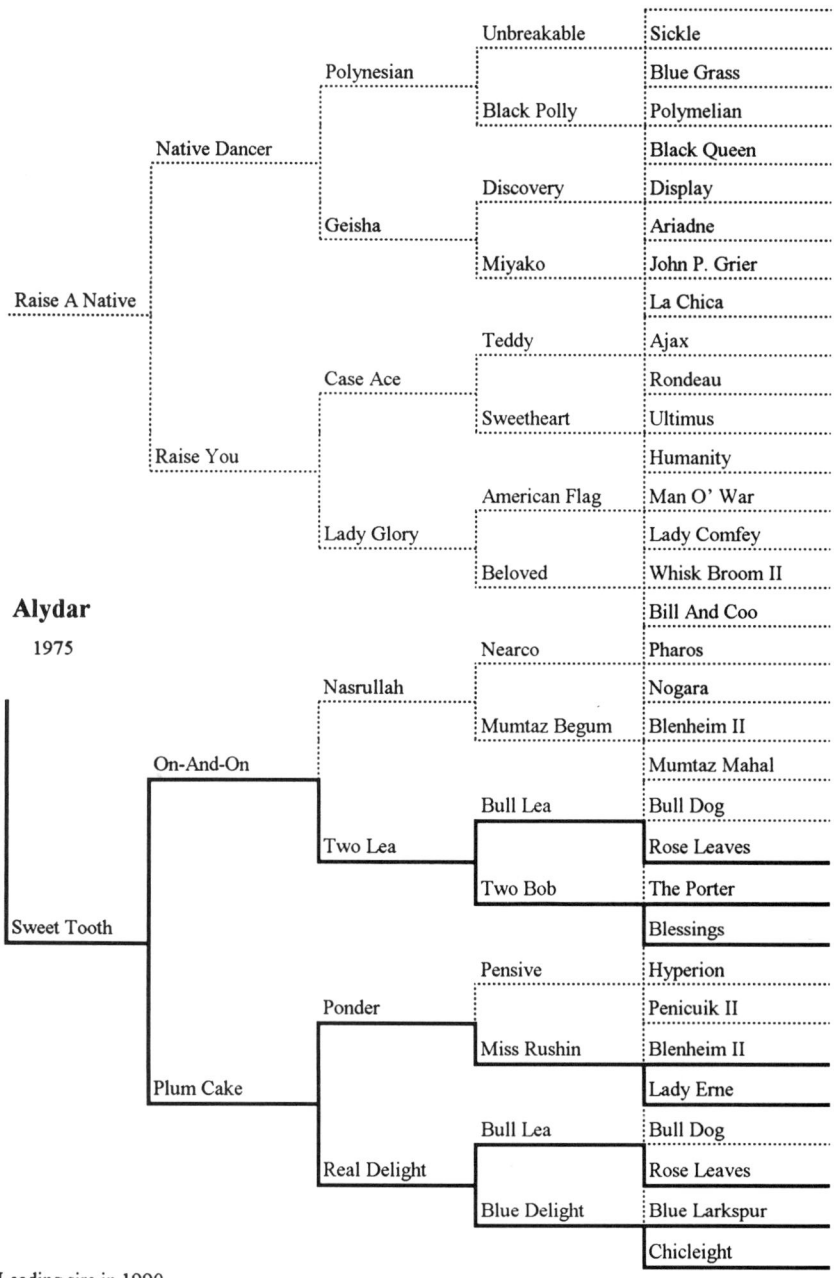

Pedigree chart:

- Raise A Native
  - Native Dancer
    - Polynesian
      - Unbreakable
        - Sickle
        - Blue Grass
      - Black Polly
        - Polymelian
        - Black Queen
    - Geisha
      - Discovery
        - Display
        - Ariadne
      - Miyako
        - John P. Grier
        - La Chica
  - Raise You
    - Case Ace
      - Teddy
        - Ajax
        - Rondeau
      - Sweetheart
        - Ultimus
        - Humanity
    - Lady Glory
      - American Flag
        - Man O' War
        - Lady Comfey
      - Beloved
        - Whisk Broom II
        - Bill And Coo

- Sweet Tooth
  - On-And-On
    - Nasrullah
      - Nearco
        - Pharos
        - Nogara
      - Mumtaz Begum
        - Blenheim II
        - Mumtaz Mahal
    - Two Lea
      - Bull Lea
        - Bull Dog
        - Rose Leaves
      - Two Bob
        - The Porter
        - Blessings
  - Plum Cake
    - Ponder
      - Pensive
        - Hyperion
        - Penicuik II
      - Miss Rushin
        - Blenheim II
        - Lady Erne
    - Real Delight
      - Bull Lea
        - Bull Dog
        - Rose Leaves
      - Blue Delight
        - Blue Larkspur
        - Chicleight

Leading sire in 1990
Sire of five Eclipse Champions: Alysheba, Criminal Type, Easy Goer, Althea and Turhona

Buckpasser
1963

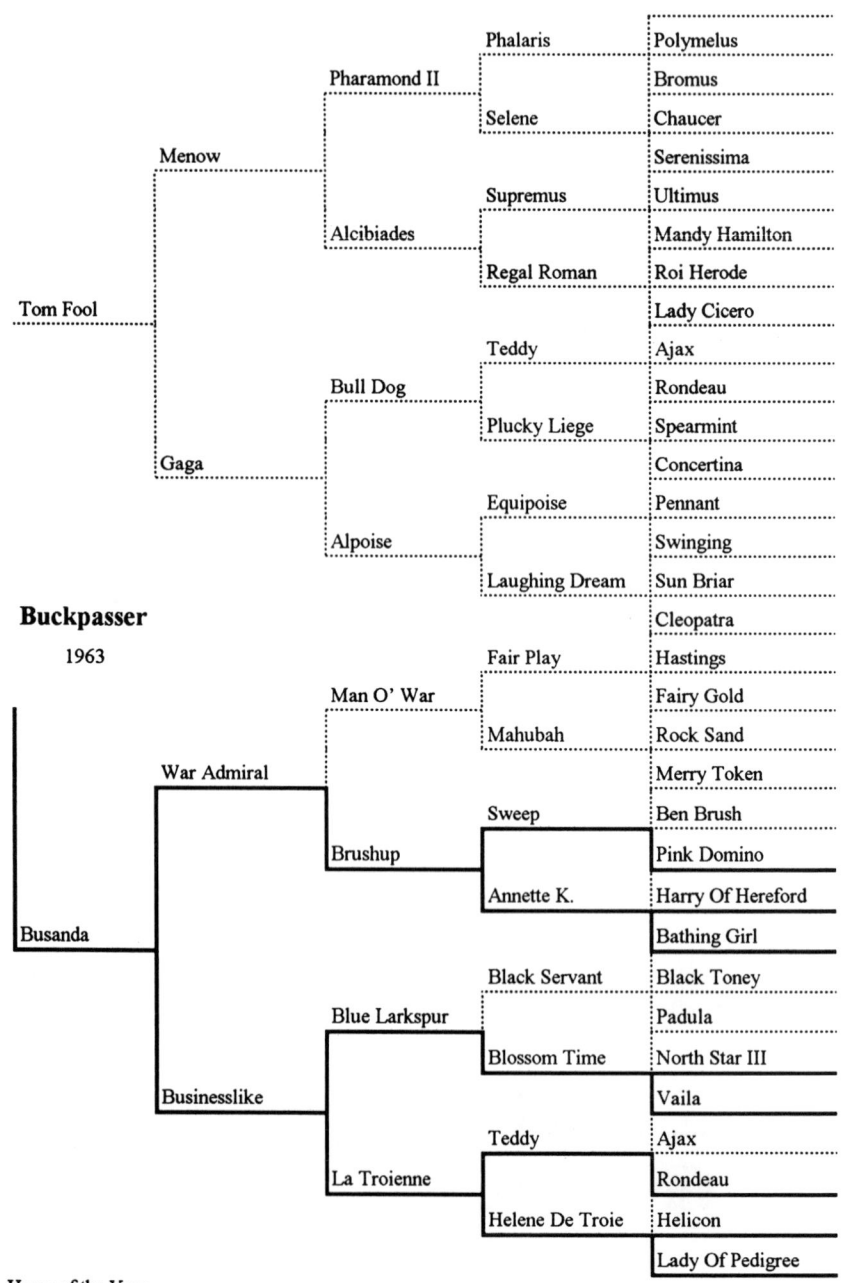

Pedigree:

- Tom Fool
  - Menow
    - Pharamond II
      - Phalaris
        - Polymelus
        - Bromus
      - Selene
        - Chaucer
        - Serenissima
    - Alcibiades
      - Supremus
        - Ultimus
        - Mandy Hamilton
      - Regal Roman
        - Roi Herode
        - Lady Cicero
  - Gaga
    - Bull Dog
      - Teddy
        - Ajax
        - Rondeau
      - Plucky Liege
        - Spearmint
        - Concertina
    - Alpoise
      - Equipoise
        - Pennant
        - Swinging
      - Laughing Dream
        - Sun Briar
        - Cleopatra
- Busanda
  - War Admiral
    - Man O' War
      - Fair Play
        - Hastings
        - Fairy Gold
      - Mahubah
        - Rock Sand
        - Merry Token
    - Brushup
      - Sweep
        - Ben Brush
        - Pink Domino
      - Annette K.
        - Harry Of Hereford
        - Bathing Girl
  - Businesslike
    - Blue Larkspur
      - Black Servant
        - Black Toney
        - Padula
      - Blossom Time
        - North Star III
        - Vaila
    - La Troienne
      - Teddy
        - Ajax
        - Rondeau
      - Helene De Troie
        - Helicon
        - Lady Of Pedigree

Horse of the Year
Champion 2- and 3-Year-Old Colt and Champion Older Male
Sire of L'Enjoleur and Norcliffe

180

Busher

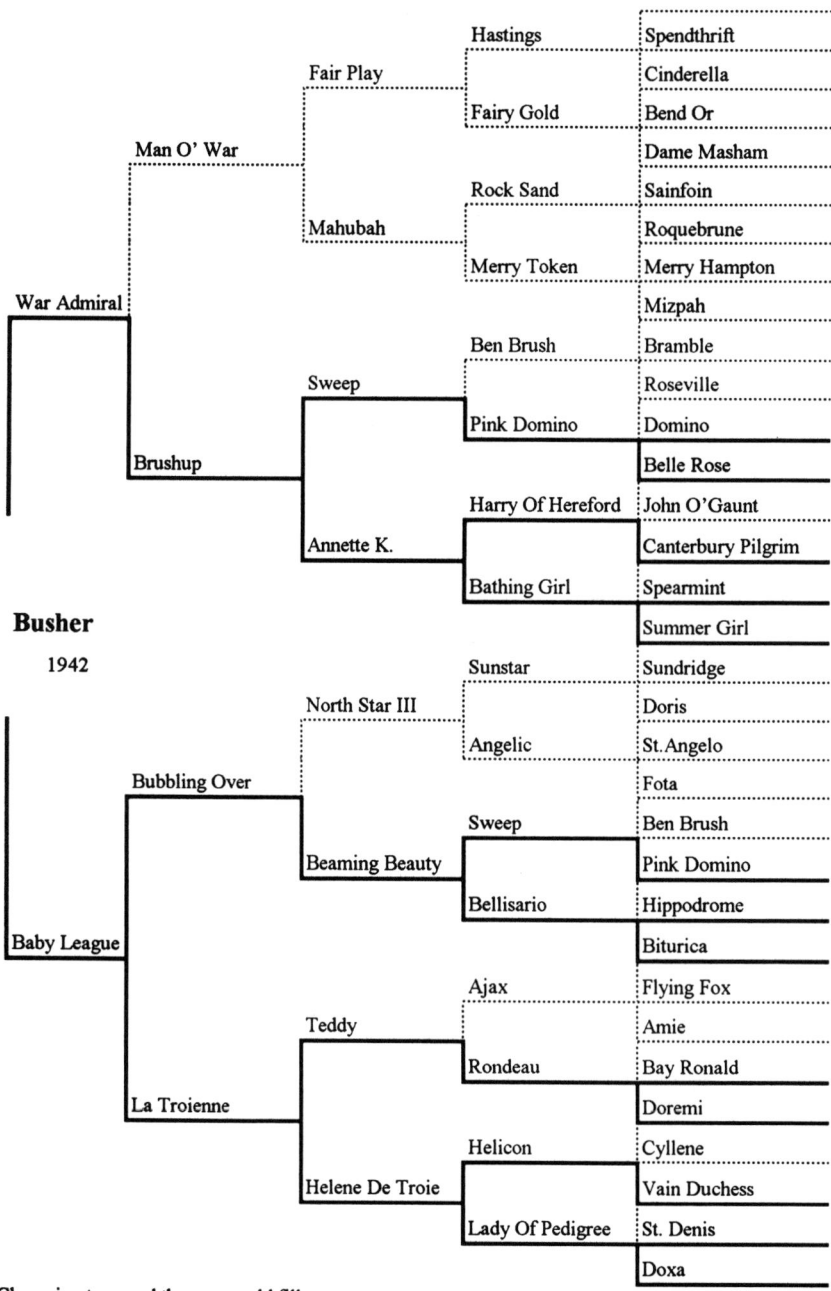

1942

Pedigree

- **War Admiral**
  - **Man O' War**
    - Fair Play
      - Hastings — Spendthrift / Cinderella
      - Fairy Gold — Bend Or / Dame Masham
    - Mahubah
      - Rock Sand — Sainfoin / Roquebrune
      - Merry Token — Merry Hampton / Mizpah
  - **Brushup**
    - Sweep
      - Ben Brush — Bramble / Roseville
      - Pink Domino — Domino / Belle Rose
    - Annette K.
      - Harry Of Hereford — John O'Gaunt / Canterbury Pilgrim
      - Bathing Girl — Spearmint / Summer Girl

- **Baby League**
  - **Bubbling Over**
    - North Star III
      - Sunstar — Sundridge / Doris
      - Angelic — St. Angelo / Fota
    - Beaming Beauty
      - Sweep — Ben Brush / Pink Domino
      - Bellisario — Hippodrome / Biturica
  - **La Troienne**
    - Teddy
      - Ajax — Flying Fox / Amie
      - Rondeau — Bay Ronald / Doremi
    - Helene De Troie
      - Helicon — Cyllene / Vain Duchess
      - Lady Of Pedigree — St. Denis / Doxa

Champion two- and three-year-old filly
1945 Horse of the Year and champion handicap mare

Citation
1945

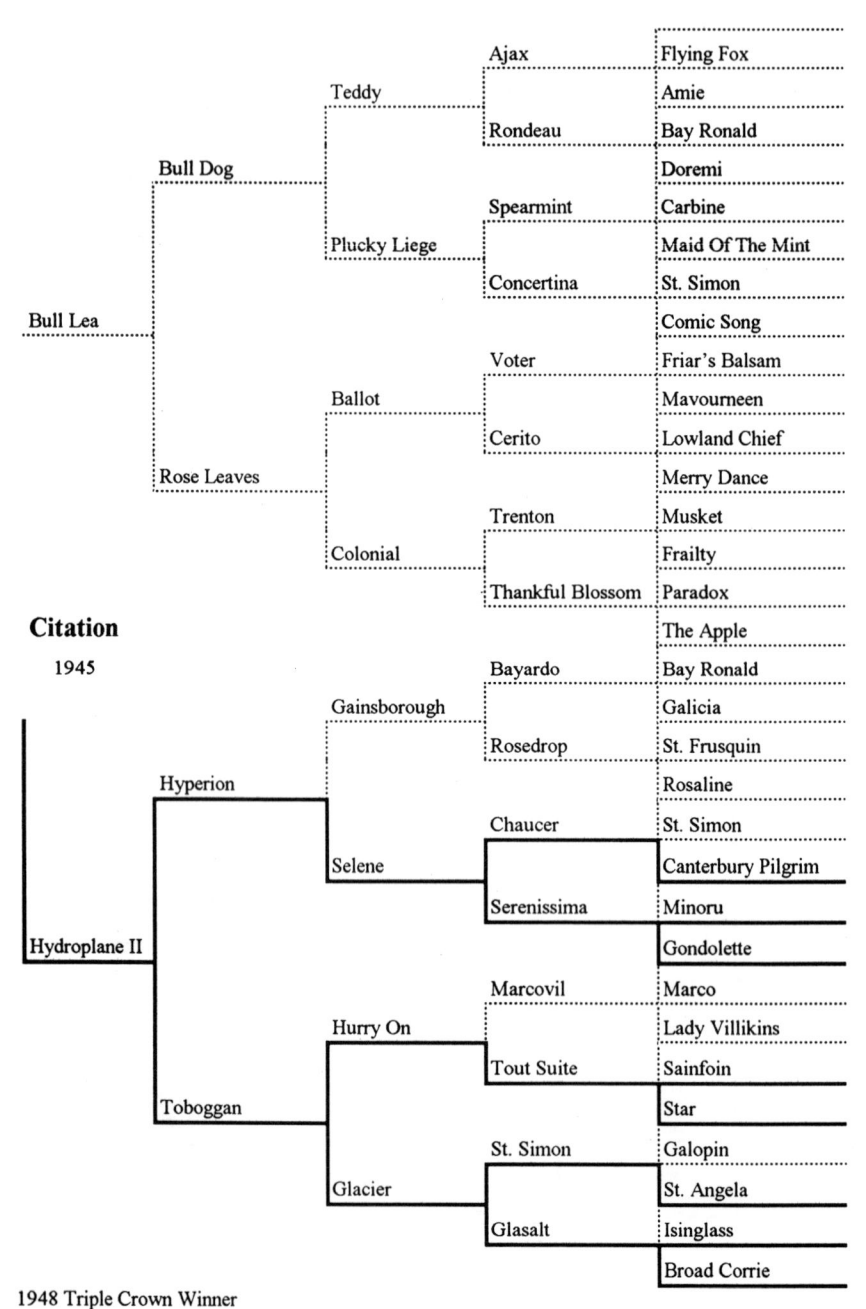

1948 Triple Crown Winner

Bull Lea	Bull Dog	Teddy	Ajax — Flying Fox
			Ajax — Amie
			Rondeau — Bay Ronald
			Rondeau — Doremi
		Plucky Liege	Spearmint — Carbine
			Spearmint — Maid Of The Mint
			Concertina — St. Simon
			Concertina — Comic Song
	Rose Leaves	Ballot	Voter — Friar's Balsam
			Voter — Mavourneen
			Cerito — Lowland Chief
			Cerito — Merry Dance
		Colonial	Trenton — Musket
			Trenton — Frailty
			Thankful Blossom — Paradox
			Thankful Blossom — The Apple
Hydroplane II	Hyperion	Gainsborough	Bayardo — Bay Ronald
			Bayardo — Galicia
			Rosedrop — St. Frusquin
			Rosedrop — Rosaline
		Selene	Chaucer — St. Simon
			Chaucer — Canterbury Pilgrim
			Serenissima — Minoru
			Serenissima — Gondolette
	Toboggan	Hurry On	Marcovil — Marco
			Marcovil — Lady Villikins
			Tout Suite — Sainfoin
			Tout Suite — Star
		Glacier	St. Simon — Galopin
			St. Simon — St. Angela
			Glasalt — Isinglass
			Glasalt — Broad Corrie

Dr. Fager
1964

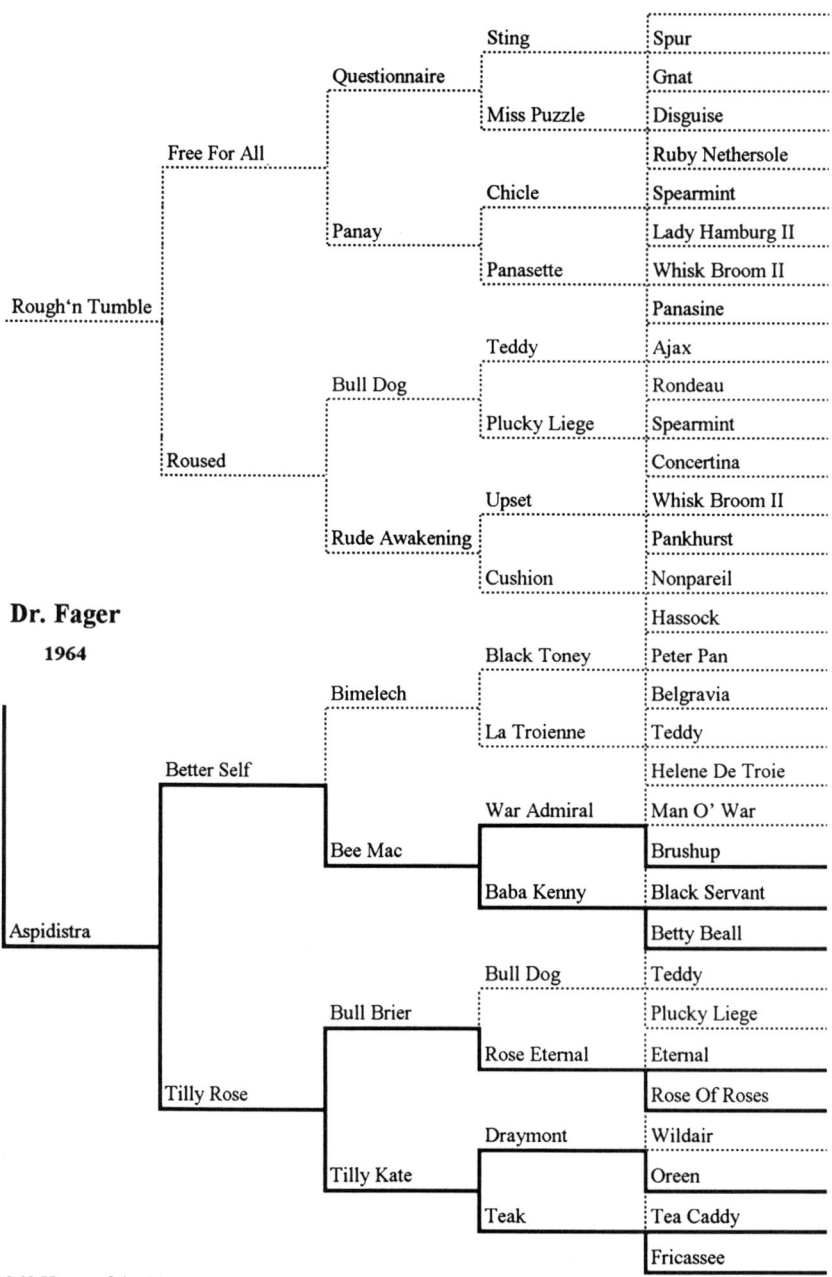

- Rough'n Tumble
  - Free For All
    - Questionnaire
      - Sting
        - Spur
        - Gnat
      - Miss Puzzle
        - Disguise
        - Ruby Nethersole
    - Panay
      - Chicle
        - Spearmint
        - Lady Hamburg II
      - Panasette
        - Whisk Broom II
        - Panasine
  - Roused
    - Bull Dog
      - Teddy
        - Ajax
        - Rondeau
      - Plucky Liege
        - Spearmint
        - Concertina
    - Rude Awakening
      - Upset
        - Whisk Broom II
        - Pankhurst
      - Cushion
        - Nonpareil
        - Hassock
- Aspidistra
  - Better Self
    - Bimelech
      - Black Toney
        - Peter Pan
        - Belgravia
      - La Troienne
        - Teddy
        - Helene De Troie
    - Bee Mac
      - War Admiral
        - Man O' War
        - Brushup
      - Baba Kenny
        - Black Servant
        - Betty Beall
  - Tilly Rose
    - Bull Brier
      - Bull Dog
        - Teddy
        - Plucky Liege
      - Rose Eternal
        - Eternal
        - Rose Of Roses
    - Tilly Kate
      - Draymont
        - Wildair
        - Oreen
      - Teak
        - Tea Caddy
        - Fricassee

1968 Horse of the Year
Champion Sprinter, Grass and Handicap
Sire of Killahoe dam of Fappiano

183

Easy Goer
1986

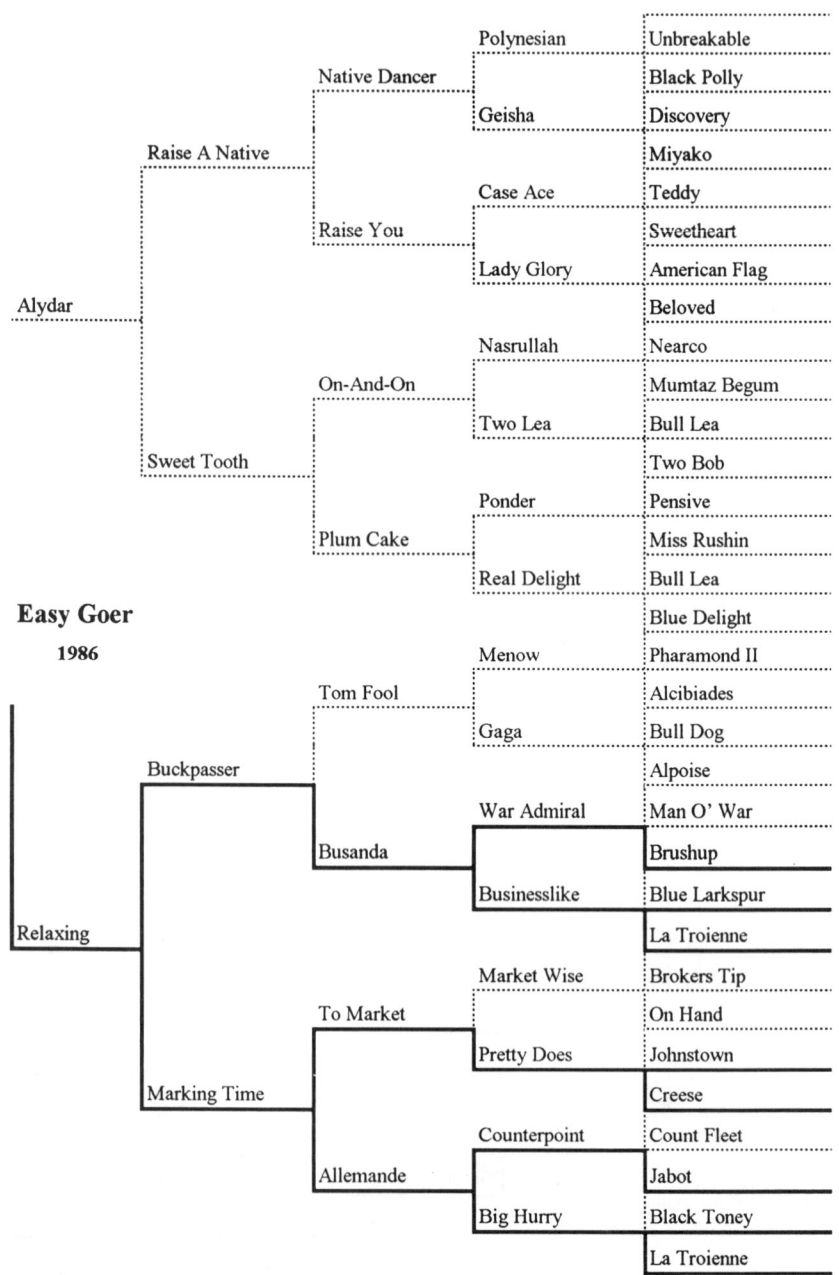

Pedigree:

- Alydar
  - Raise A Native
    - Native Dancer
      - Polynesian
        - Unbreakable
        - Black Polly
      - Geisha
        - Discovery
        - Miyako
    - Raise You
      - Case Ace
        - Teddy
        - Sweetheart
      - Lady Glory
        - American Flag
        - Beloved
  - Sweet Tooth
    - On-And-On
      - Nasrullah
        - Nearco
        - Mumtaz Begum
      - Two Lea
        - Bull Lea
        - Two Bob
    - Plum Cake
      - Ponder
        - Pensive
        - Miss Rushin
      - Real Delight
        - Bull Lea
        - Blue Delight
- Relaxing
  - Buckpasser
    - Tom Fool
      - Menow
        - Pharamond II
        - Alcibiades
      - Gaga
        - Bull Dog
        - Alpoise
    - Busanda
      - War Admiral
        - Man O' War
        - Brushup
      - Businesslike
        - Blue Larkspur
        - La Troienne
  - Marking Time
    - To Market
      - Market Wise
        - Brokers Tip
        - On Hand
      - Pretty Does
        - Johnstown
        - Creese
    - Allemande
      - Counterpoint
        - Count Fleet
        - Jabot
      - Big Hurry
        - Black Toney
        - La Troienne

Champion Two-Year-Old and Classic Winner:
Belmont Stakes, Jockey Club Gold Cup, Travers Stakes, Woodward Stakes
Earned $4,873,770
Sire of champion, My Flag

Grey Dawn II
1962

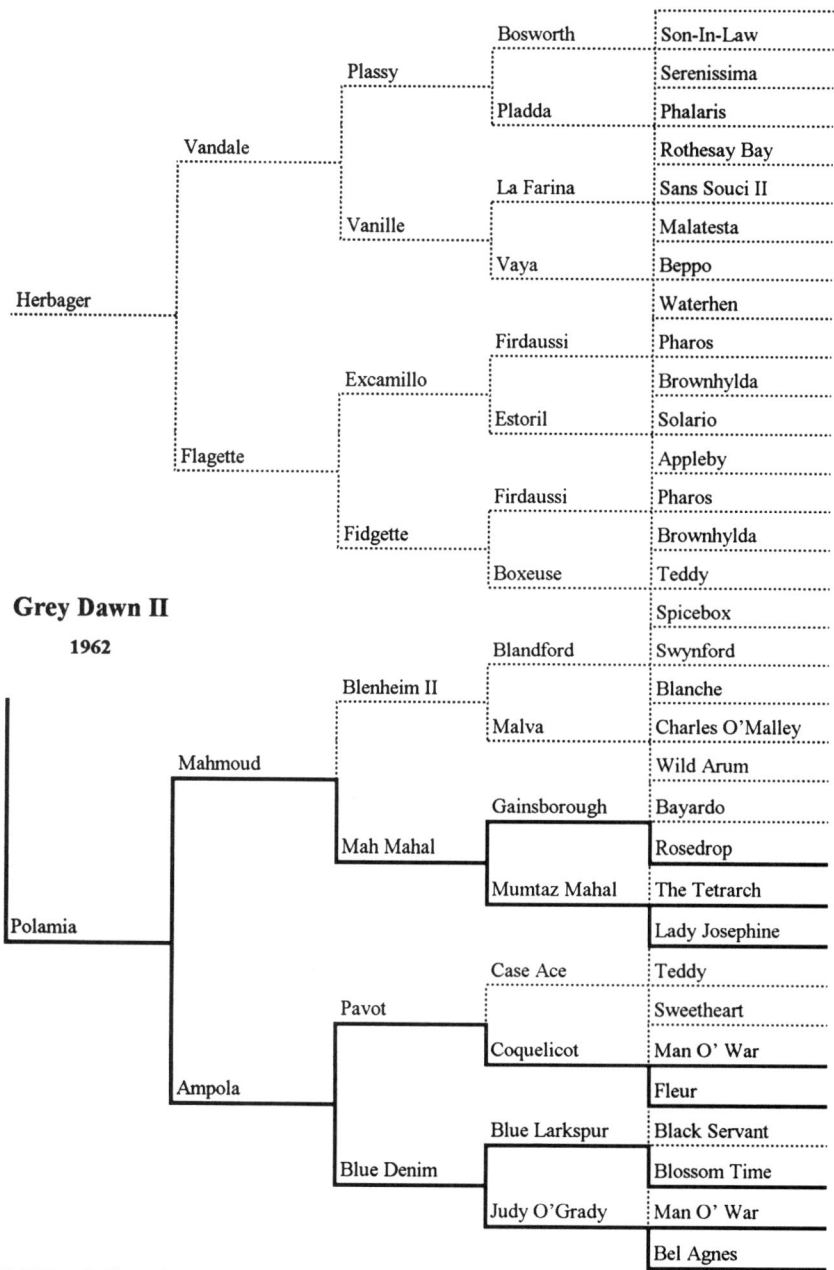

Herbager
- Vandale
  - Plassy
    - Bosworth
      - Son-In-Law
      - Serenissima
    - Pladda
      - Phalaris
      - Rothesay Bay
  - Vanille
    - La Farina
      - Sans Souci II
      - Malatesta
    - Vaya
      - Beppo
      - Waterhen
- Flagette
  - Excamillo
    - Firdaussi
      - Pharos
      - Brownhylda
    - Estoril
      - Solario
      - Appleby
  - Fidgette
    - Firdaussi
      - Pharos
      - Brownhylda
    - Boxeuse
      - Teddy
      - Spicebox

Polamia
- Mahmoud
  - Blenheim II
    - Blandford
      - Swynford
      - Blanche
    - Malva
      - Charles O'Malley
      - Wild Arum
  - Mah Mahal
    - Gainsborough
      - Bayardo
      - Rosedrop
    - Mumtaz Mahal
      - The Tetrarch
      - Lady Josephine
- Ampola
  - Pavot
    - Case Ace
      - Teddy
      - Sweetheart
    - Coquelicot
      - Man O' War
      - Fleur
  - Blue Denim
    - Blue Larkspur
      - Black Servant
      - Blossom Time
    - Judy O'Grady
      - Man O' War
      - Bel Agnes

1964 French Champion Two-Year-Old

Northern Dancer
1961

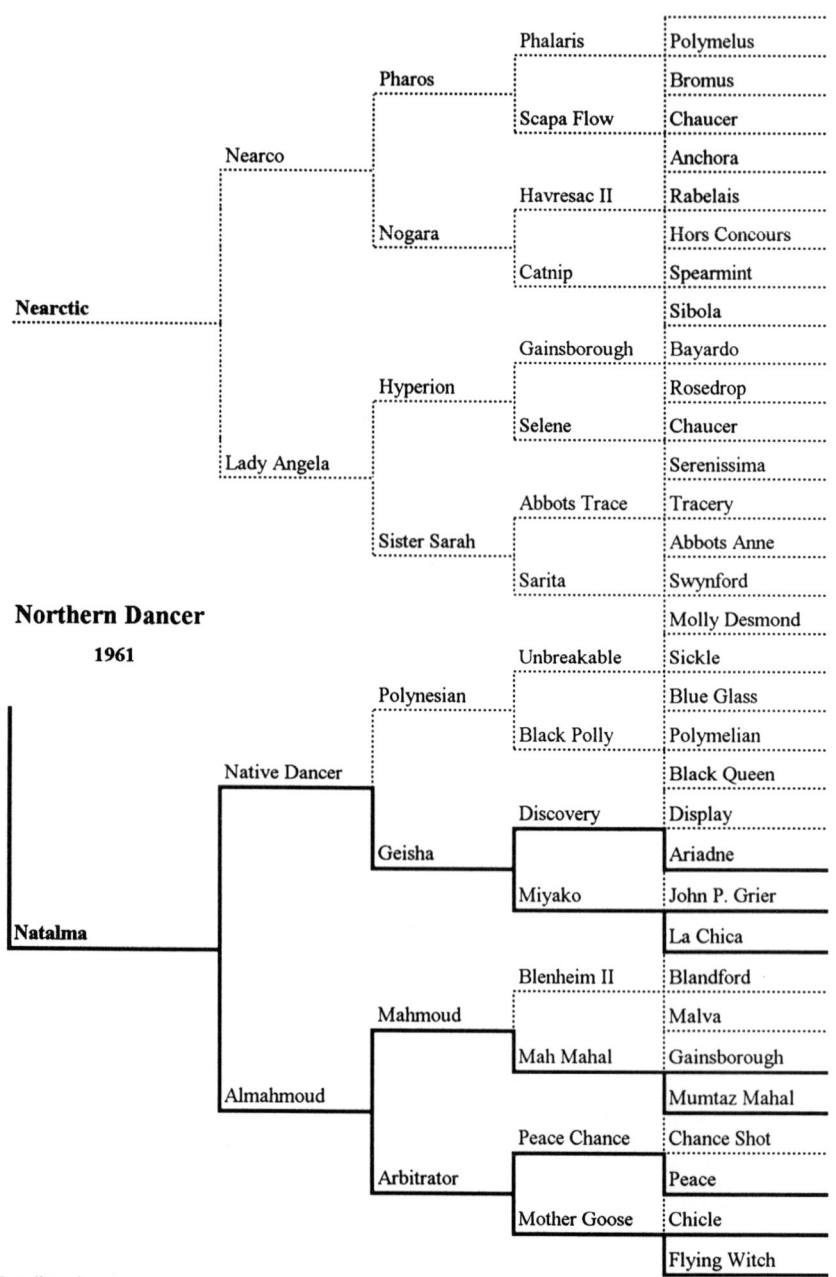

Nearctic	Nearco	Pharos	Phalaris	Polymelus
				Bromus
			Scapa Flow	Chaucer
				Anchora
		Nogara	Havresac II	Rabelais
				Hors Concours
			Catnip	Spearmint
				Sibola
	Lady Angela	Hyperion	Gainsborough	Bayardo
				Rosedrop
			Selene	Chaucer
				Serenissima
		Sister Sarah	Abbots Trace	Tracery
				Abbots Anne
			Sarita	Swynford
				Molly Desmond
Natalma	Native Dancer	Polynesian	Unbreakable	Sickle
				Blue Glass
			Black Polly	Polymelian
				Black Queen
		Geisha	Discovery	Display
				Ariadne
			Miyako	John P. Grier
				La Chica
	Almahmoud	Mahmoud	Blenheim II	Blandford
				Malva
			Mah Mahal	Gainsborough
				Mumtaz Mahal
		Arbitrator	Peace Chance	Chance Shot
				Peace
			Mother Goose	Chicle
				Flying Witch

Leading sire
One of the most influential sires of the 20th century
Sire of 146 stakes winners (23%) including 24 champions

186

Nureyev
1977

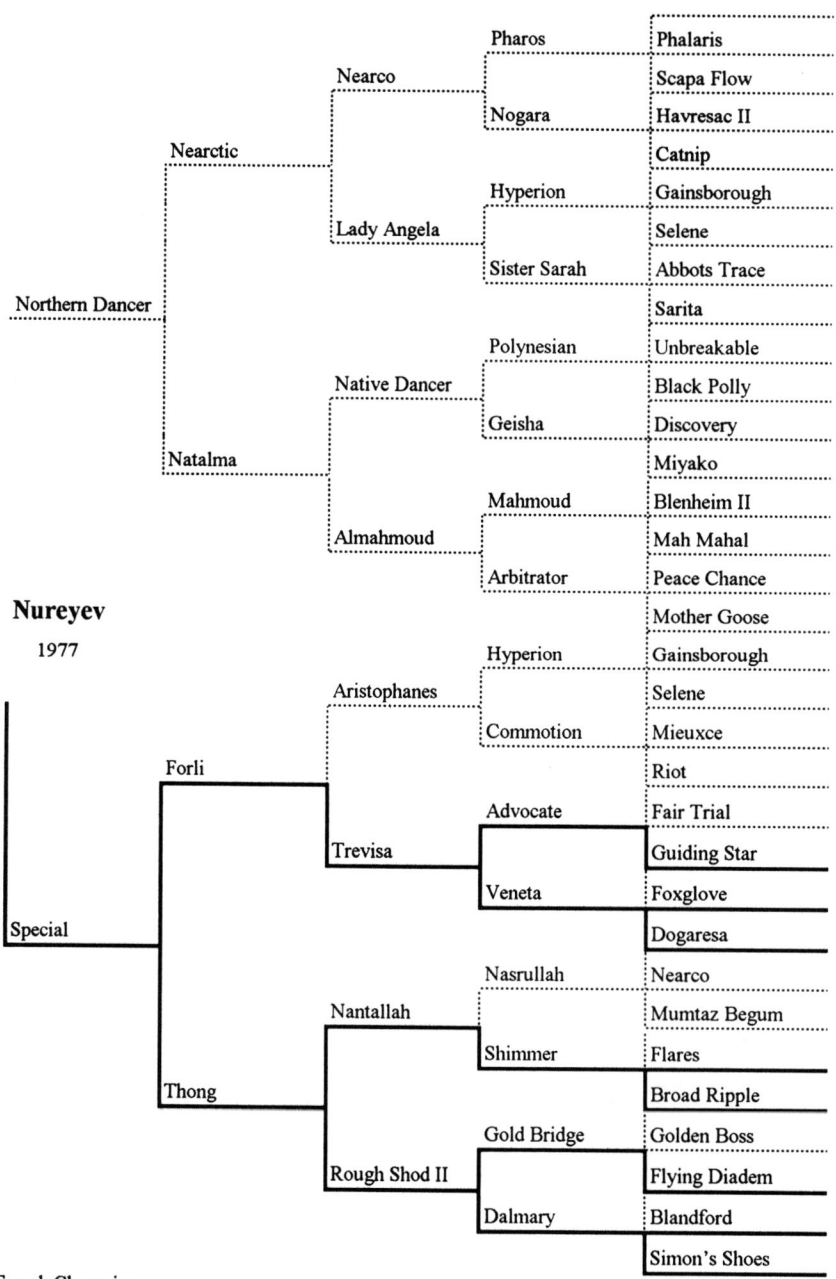

```
                                            ┌─ Pharos ──────┬─ Phalaris
                              ┌─ Nearco ────┤               └─ Scapa Flow
                              │             └─ Nogara ──────┬─ Havresac II
              ┌─ Nearctic ────┤                             └─ Catnip
              │               │             ┌─ Hyperion ────┬─ Gainsborough
              │               └─ Lady Angela┤               └─ Selene
              │                             └─ Sister Sarah ┬─ Abbots Trace
Northern Dancer┤                                            └─ Sarita
              │                             ┌─ Polynesian ──┬─ Unbreakable
              │               ┌─ Native Dancer              └─ Black Polly
              │               │             └─ Geisha ──────┬─ Discovery
              └─ Natalma ─────┤                             └─ Miyako
                              │             ┌─ Mahmoud ─────┬─ Blenheim II
                              └─ Almahmoud ─┤               └─ Mah Mahal
                                            └─ Arbitrator ──┬─ Peace Chance
                                                            └─ Mother Goose

                                            ┌─ Hyperion ────┬─ Gainsborough
                              ┌─ Aristophanes               └─ Selene
              ┌─ Forli ───────┤             └─ Commotion ───┬─ Mieuxce
              │               │                             └─ Riot
              │               │             ┌─ Advocate ────┬─ Fair Trial
              │               └─ Trevisa ───┤               └─ Guiding Star
              │                             └─ Veneta ──────┬─ Foxglove
Special ──────┤                                             └─ Dogaresa
              │                             ┌─ Nasrullah ───┬─ Nearco
              │               ┌─ Nantallah ─┤               └─ Mumtaz Begum
              │               │             └─ Shimmer ─────┬─ Flares
              └─ Thong ───────┤                             └─ Broad Ripple
                              │             ┌─ Gold Bridge ─┬─ Golden Boss
                              └─ Rough Shod II              └─ Flying Diadem
                                            └─ Dalmary ─────┬─ Blandford
                                                            └─ Simon's Shoes
```

French Champion
Sire of 16 champions including multiple champion, Miesque

Omaha
1932

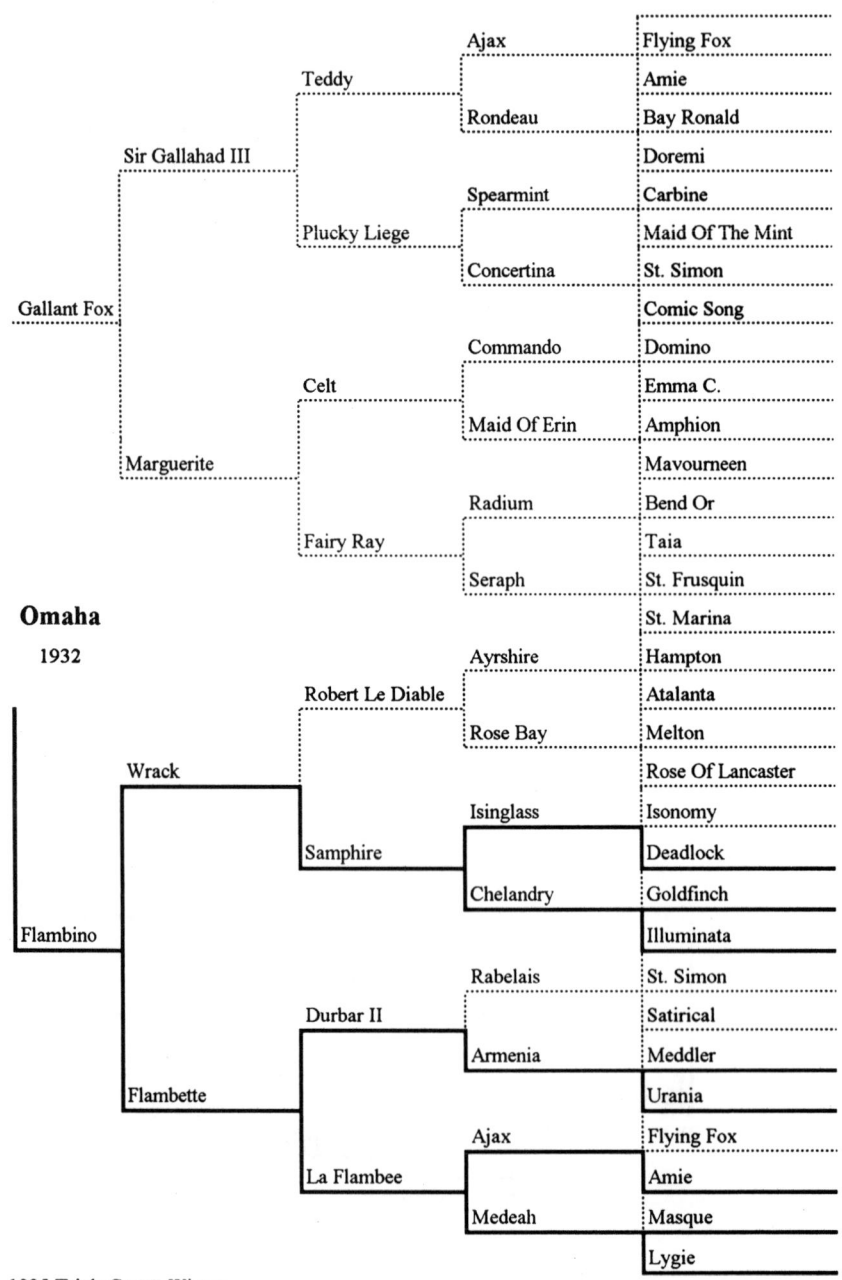

1935 Triple Crown Winner

- Gallant Fox
  - Sir Gallahad III
    - Teddy
      - Ajax
        - Flying Fox
        - Amie
      - Rondeau
        - Bay Ronald
        - Doremi
    - Plucky Liege
      - Spearmint
        - Carbine
        - Maid Of The Mint
      - Concertina
        - St. Simon
        - Comic Song
  - Marguerite
    - Celt
      - Commando
        - Domino
        - Emma C.
      - Maid Of Erin
        - Amphion
        - Mavourneen
    - Fairy Ray
      - Radium
        - Bend Or
        - Taia
      - Seraph
        - St. Frusquin
        - St. Marina
- Flambino
  - Wrack
    - Robert Le Diable
      - Ayrshire
        - Hampton
        - Atalanta
      - Rose Bay
        - Melton
        - Rose Of Lancaster
    - Samphire
      - Isinglass
        - Isonomy
        - Deadlock
      - Chelandry
        - Goldfinch
        - Illuminata
  - Flambette
    - Durbar II
      - Rabelais
        - St. Simon
        - Satirical
      - Armenia
        - Meddler
        - Urania
    - La Flambee
      - Ajax
        - Flying Fox
        - Amie
      - Medeah
        - Masque
        - Lygie

188

Prince John
1953

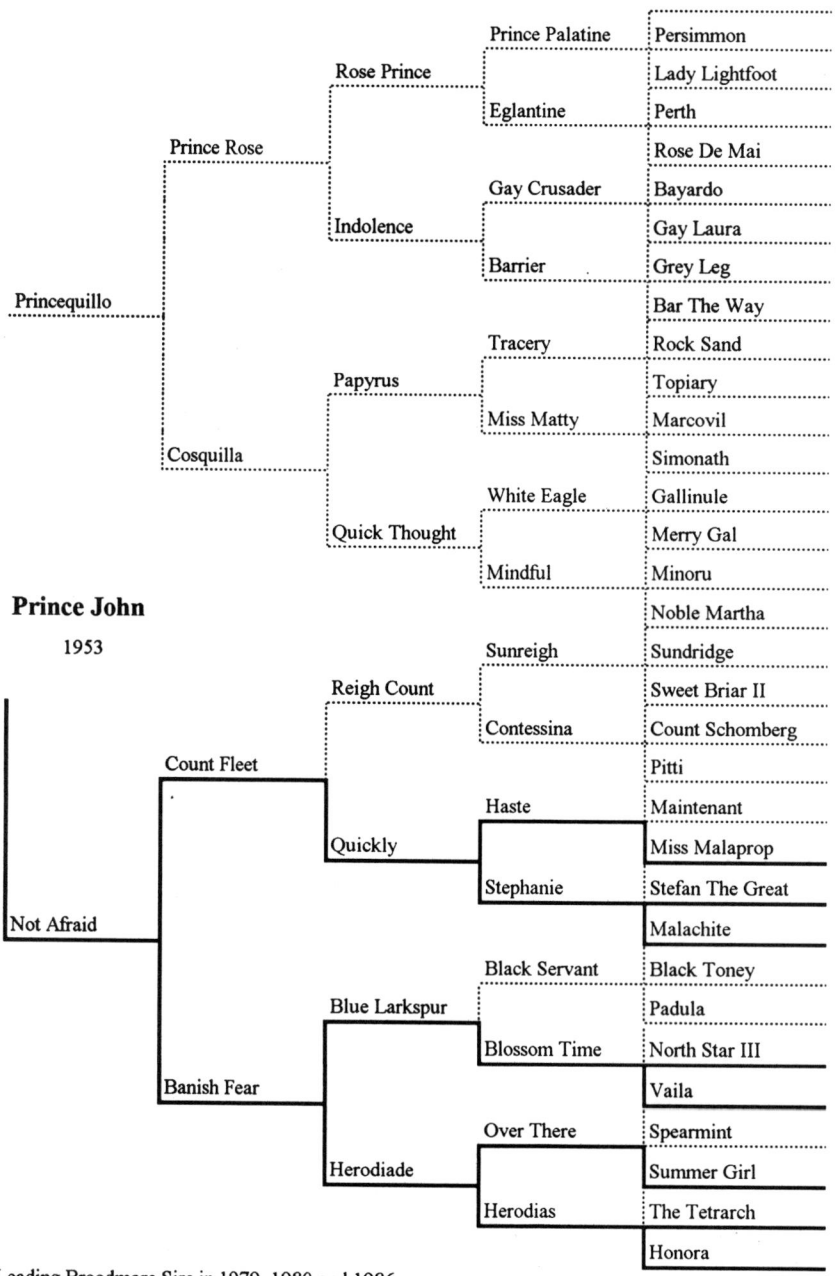

```
Princequillo ─┬─ Prince Rose ─┬─ Rose Prince ──┬─ Prince Palatine ─┬─ Persimmon
              │               │                │                   └─ Lady Lightfoot
              │               │                └─ Eglantine ──────┬─ Perth
              │               │                                    └─ Rose De Mai
              │               └─ Indolence ────┬─ Gay Crusader ───┬─ Bayardo
              │                                │                   └─ Gay Laura
              │                                └─ Barrier ────────┬─ Grey Leg
              │                                                    └─ Bar The Way
              └─ Cosquilla ───┬─ Papyrus ──────┬─ Tracery ────────┬─ Rock Sand
                              │                │                   └─ Topiary
                              │                └─ Miss Matty ─────┬─ Marcovil
                              │                                    └─ Simonath
                              └─ Quick Thought ┬─ White Eagle ────┬─ Gallinule
                                               │                   └─ Merry Gal
                                               └─ Mindful ────────┬─ Minoru
                                                                   └─ Noble Martha

Not Afraid ─┬─ Count Fleet ──┬─ Reigh Count ──┬─ Sunreigh ───────┬─ Sundridge
            │                │                │                   └─ Sweet Briar II
            │                │                └─ Contessina ─────┬─ Count Schomberg
            │                │                                    └─ Pitti
            │                └─ Quickly ──────┬─ Haste ──────────┬─ Maintenant
            │                                 │                   └─ Miss Malaprop
            │                                 └─ Stephanie ──────┬─ Stefan The Great
            │                                                     └─ Malachite
            └─ Banish Fear ──┬─ Blue Larkspur ┬─ Black Servant ──┬─ Black Toney
                             │                │                   └─ Padula
                             │                └─ Blossom Time ───┬─ North Star III
                             │                                    └─ Vaila
                             └─ Herodiade ────┬─ Over There ─────┬─ Spearmint
                                              │                   └─ Summer Girl
                                              └─ Herodias ───────┬─ The Tetrarch
                                                                  └─ Honora
```

Leading Broodmare Sire in 1979, 1980 and 1986
Broodmare sire of Alleged, Cozzene, Riverman and Palace Music

Seeking The Gold
1985

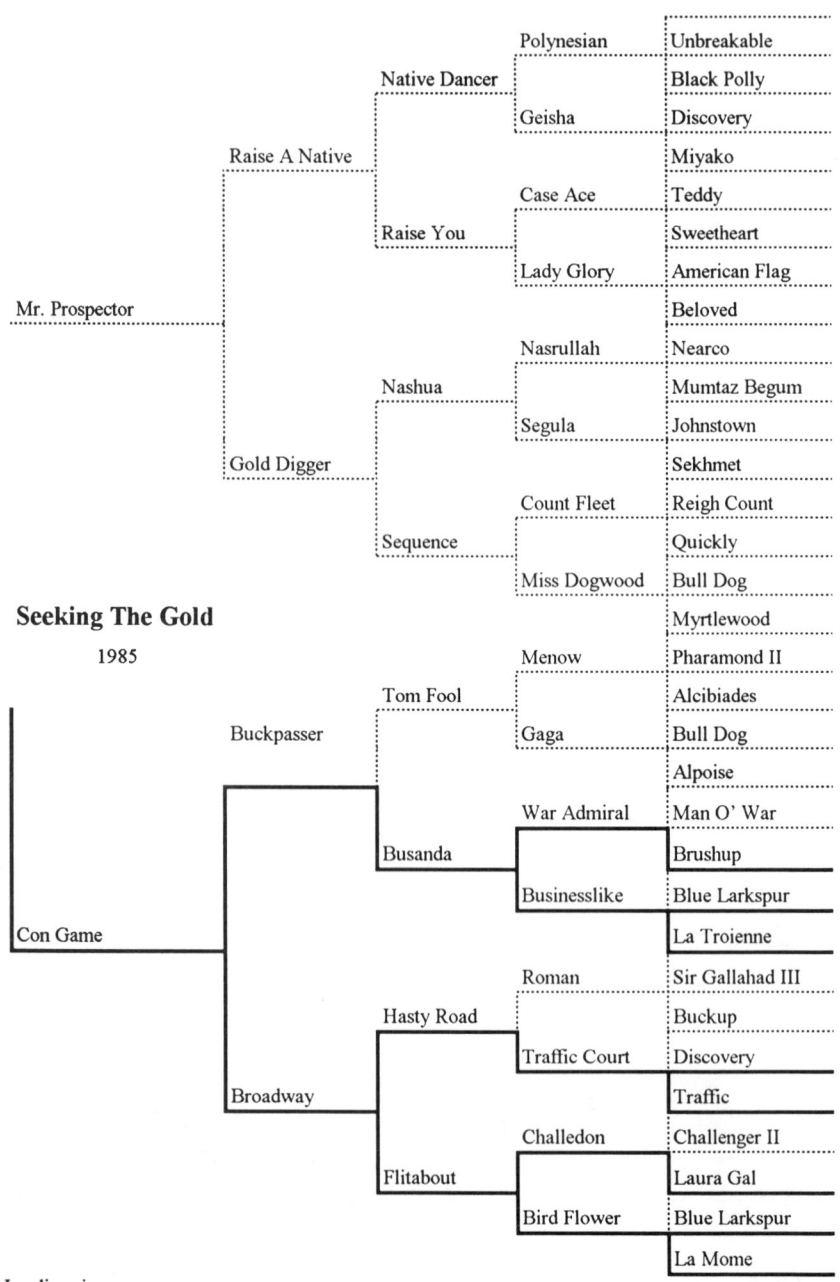

```
                                                 ┌─ Polynesian      ┌─ Unbreakable
                              ┌─ Native Dancer ──┤                  └─ Black Polly
                              │                  └─ Geisha          ┌─ Discovery
              ┌─ Raise A Native ─┤                                  └─ Miyako
              │               │                  ┌─ Case Ace        ┌─ Teddy
              │               └─ Raise You ──────┤                  └─ Sweetheart
              │                                  └─ Lady Glory      ┌─ American Flag
Mr. Prospector ─┤                                                   └─ Beloved
              │                                  ┌─ Nasrullah       ┌─ Nearco
              │               ┌─ Nashua ─────────┤                  └─ Mumtaz Begum
              │               │                  └─ Segula          ┌─ Johnstown
              └─ Gold Digger ─┤                                     └─ Sekhmet
                              │                  ┌─ Count Fleet     ┌─ Reigh Count
                              └─ Sequence ───────┤                  └─ Quickly
                                                 └─ Miss Dogwood    ┌─ Bull Dog
                                                                    └─ Myrtlewood

                                                 ┌─ Menow           ┌─ Pharamond II
                              ┌─ Tom Fool ───────┤                  └─ Alcibiades
                              │                  └─ Gaga            ┌─ Bull Dog
              ┌─ Buckpasser ──┤                                     └─ Alpoise
              │               │                  ┌─ War Admiral     ┌─ Man O' War
              │               └─ Busanda ────────┤                  └─ Brushup
              │                                  └─ Businesslike    ┌─ Blue Larkspur
Con Game ─────┤                                                     └─ La Troienne
              │                                  ┌─ Roman           ┌─ Sir Gallahad III
              │               ┌─ Hasty Road ─────┤                  └─ Buckup
              │               │                  └─ Traffic Court   ┌─ Discovery
              └─ Broadway ────┤                                     └─ Traffic
                              │                  ┌─ Challedon       ┌─ Challenger II
                              └─ Flitabout ──────┤                  └─ Laura Gal
                                                 └─ Bird Flower     ┌─ Blue Larkspur
                                                                    └─ La Mome
```

Leading sire
Earned more than 2.3 million

Sir Gallahad III
1920

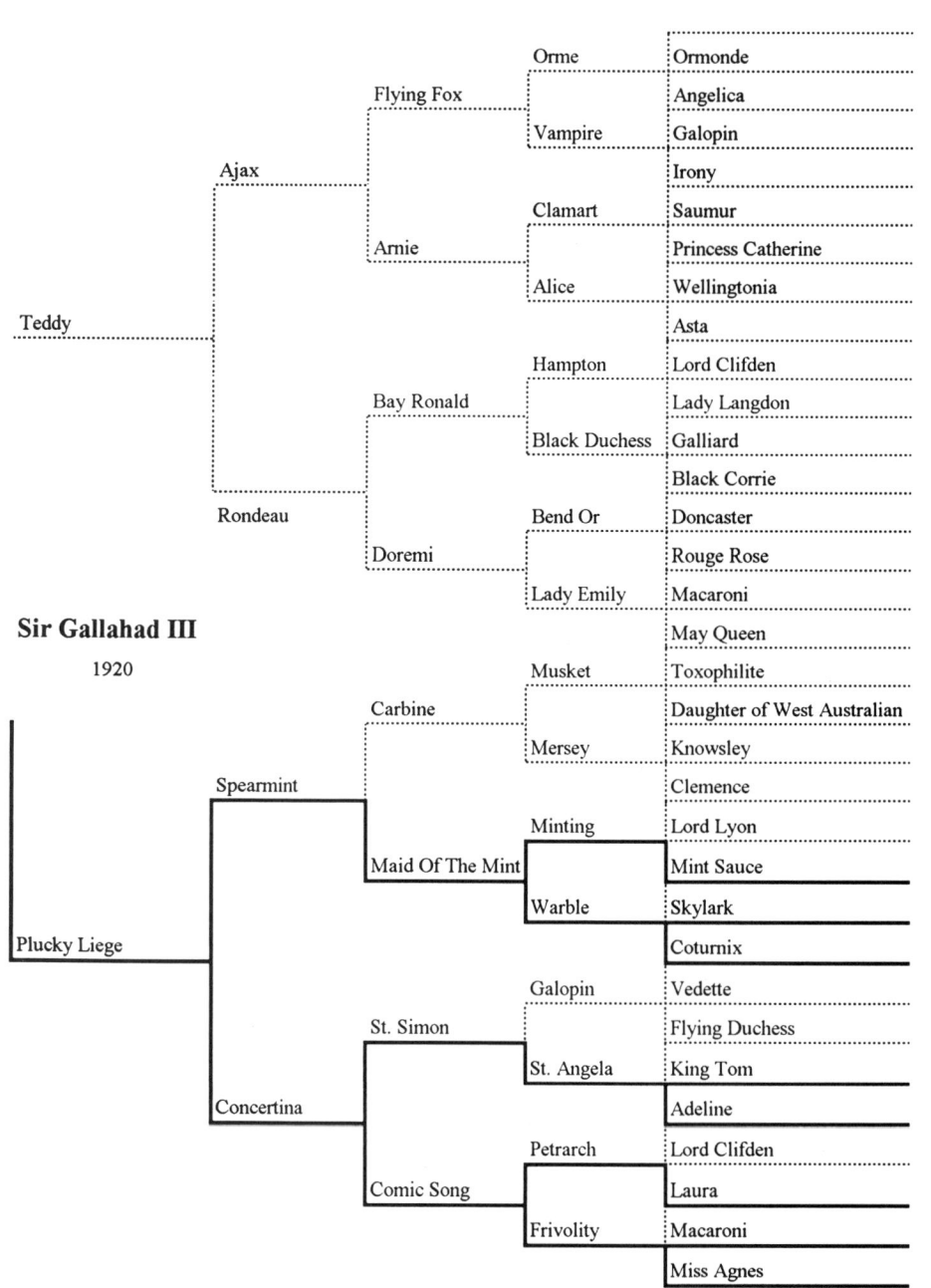

Teddy
- Ajax
  - Flying Fox
    - Orme
      - Ormonde
      - Angelica
    - Vampire
      - Galopin
      - Irony
  - Arnie
    - Clamart
      - Saumur
      - Princess Catherine
    - Alice
      - Wellingtonia
      - Asta
- Rondeau
  - Bay Ronald
    - Hampton
      - Lord Clifden
      - Lady Langdon
    - Black Duchess
      - Galliard
      - Black Corrie
  - Doremi
    - Bend Or
      - Doncaster
      - Rouge Rose
    - Lady Emily
      - Macaroni
      - May Queen

Plucky Liege
- Spearmint
  - Carbine
    - Musket
      - Toxophilite
      - Daughter of West Australian
    - Mersey
      - Knowsley
      - Clemence
  - Maid Of The Mint
    - Minting
      - Lord Lyon
      - Mint Sauce
    - Warble
      - Skylark
      - Coturnix
- Concertina
  - St. Simon
    - Galopin
      - Vedette
      - Flying Duchess
    - St. Angela
      - King Tom
      - Adeline
  - Comic Song
    - Petrarch
      - Lord Clifden
      - Laura
    - Frivolity
      - Macaroni
      - Miss Agnes

One of America's greatest broodmare sires
Sir Gallahad III was the leading sire of broodmares for 12 years
Ranked among the top 20 of leading sires of broodmares for 24 consecutive years

Somethingroyal
1952

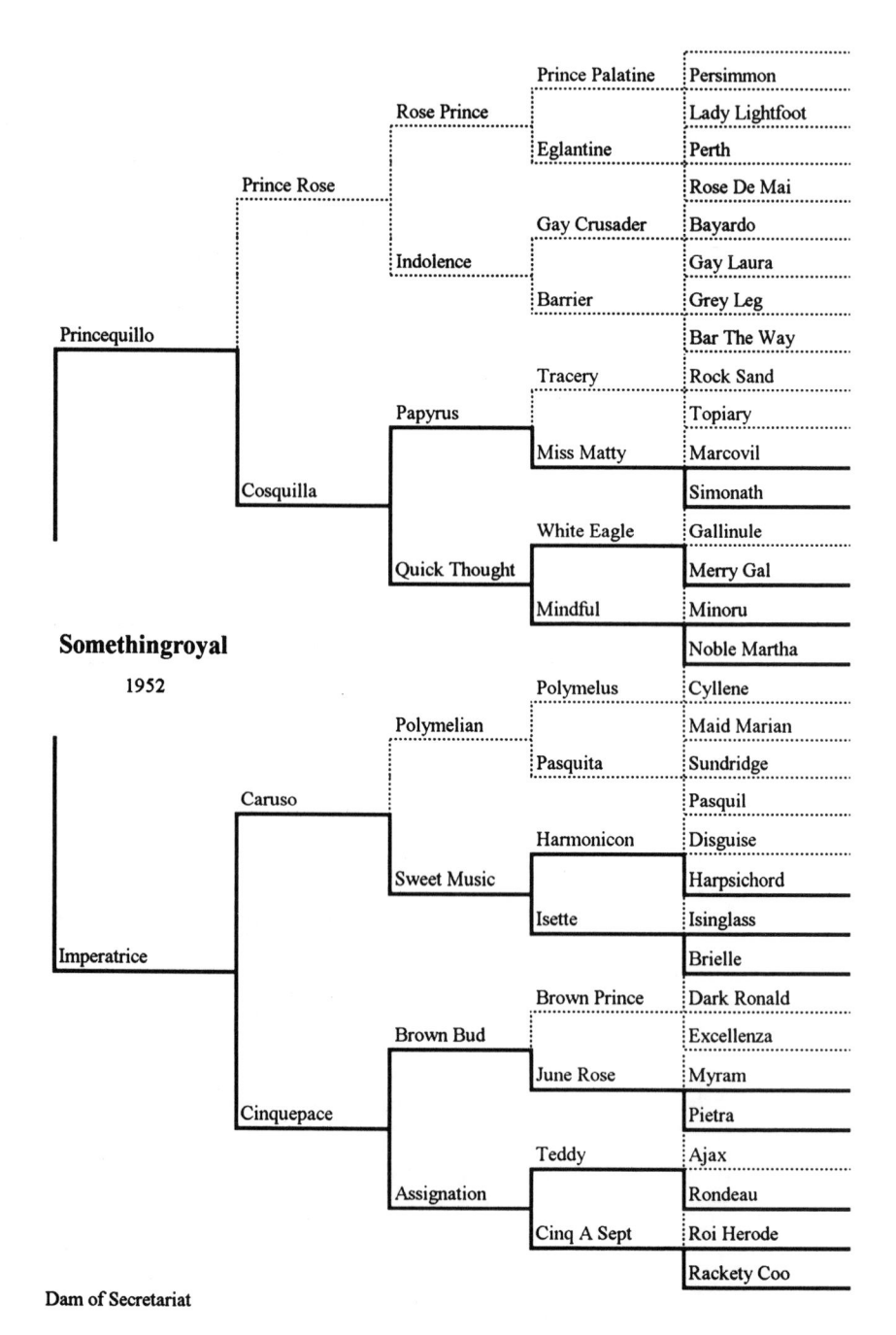

Dam of Secretariat

Generation 1	Generation 2	Generation 3	Generation 4	Generation 5
Princequillo	Prince Rose	Rose Prince	Prince Palatine	Persimmon
				Lady Lightfoot
			Eglantine	Perth
				Rose De Mai
		Indolence	Gay Crusader	Bayardo
				Gay Laura
			Barrier	Grey Leg
				Bar The Way
	Cosquilla	Papyrus	Tracery	Rock Sand
				Topiary
			Miss Matty	Marcovil
				Simonath
		Quick Thought	White Eagle	Gallinule
				Merry Gal
			Mindful	Minoru
				Noble Martha
Imperatrice	Caruso	Polymelian	Polymelus	Cyllene
				Maid Marian
			Pasquita	Sundridge
				Pasquil
		Sweet Music	Harmonicon	Disguise
				Harpsichord
			Isette	Isinglass
				Brielle
	Cinquepace	Brown Bud	Brown Prince	Dark Ronald
				Excellenza
			June Rose	Myram
				Pietra
		Assignation	Teddy	Ajax
				Rondeau
			Cinq A Sept	Roi Herode
				Rackety Coo

Soviet Problem
1990

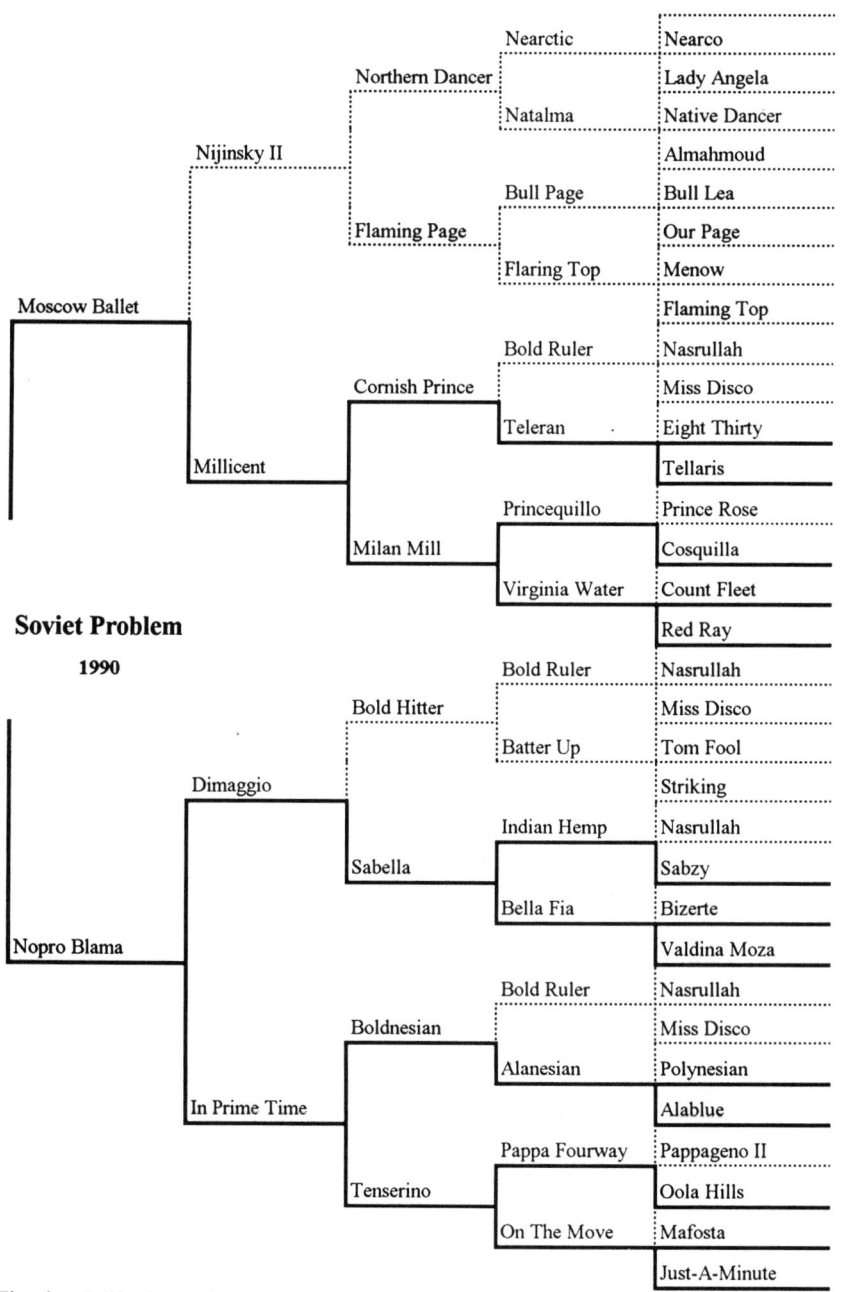

Moscow Ballet
- Nijinsky II
  - Northern Dancer
    - Nearctic
      - Nearco
      - Lady Angela
    - Natalma
      - Native Dancer
      - Almahmoud
  - Flaming Page
    - Bull Page
      - Bull Lea
      - Our Page
    - Flaring Top
      - Menow
      - Flaming Top
- Millicent
  - Cornish Prince
    - Bold Ruler
      - Nasrullah
      - Miss Disco
    - Teleran
      - Eight Thirty
      - Tellaris
  - Milan Mill
    - Princequillo
      - Prince Rose
      - Cosquilla
    - Virginia Water
      - Count Fleet
      - Red Ray

Nopro Blama
- Dimaggio
  - Bold Hitter
    - Bold Ruler
      - Nasrullah
      - Miss Disco
    - Batter Up
      - Tom Fool
      - Striking
  - Sabella
    - Indian Hemp
      - Nasrullah
      - Sabzy
    - Bella Fia
      - Bizerte
      - Valdina Moza
- In Prime Time
  - Boldnesian
    - Bold Ruler
      - Nasrullah
      - Miss Disco
    - Alanesian
      - Polynesian
      - Alablue
  - Tenserino
    - Pappa Fourway
      - Pappageno II
      - Oola Hills
    - On The Move
      - Mafosta
      - Just-A-Minute

First time California bred four-time champion
   1994 Horse of the Year, Sprint, Turf and Older mare
1994 High Weight Filly
Earned more than $900,000

St. Simon
1881

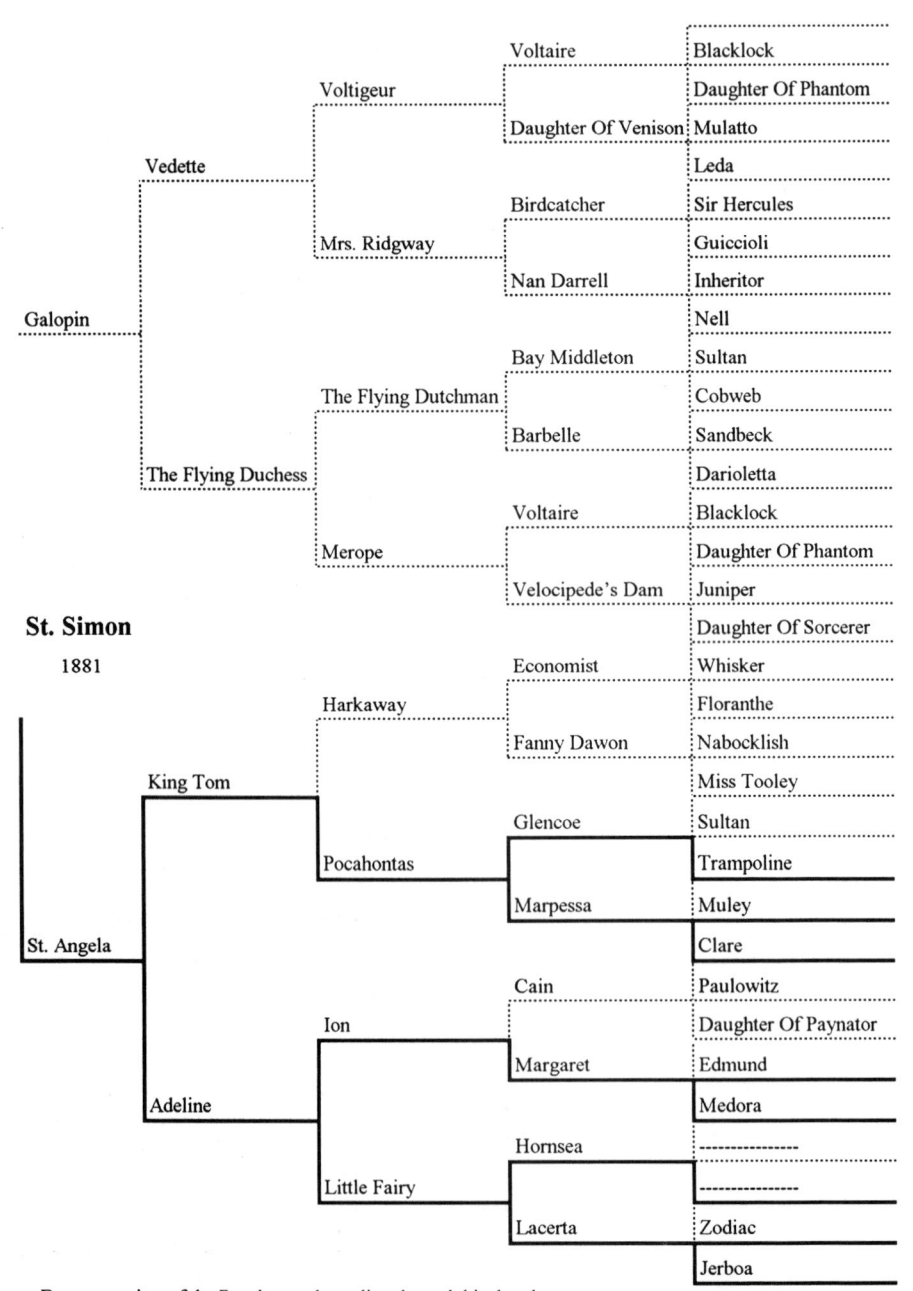

Galopin	Vedette	Voltigeur	Voltaire	Blacklock
				Daughter Of Phantom
			Daughter Of Venison	Mulatto
				Leda
		Mrs. Ridgway	Birdcatcher	Sir Hercules
				Guiccioli
			Nan Darrell	Inheritor
				Nell
	The Flying Duchess	The Flying Dutchman	Bay Middleton	Sultan
				Cobweb
			Barbelle	Sandbeck
				Darioletta
		Merope	Voltaire	Blacklock
				Daughter Of Phantom
			Velocipede's Dam	Juniper
				Daughter Of Sorcerer
St. Angela	King Tom	Harkaway	Economist	Whisker
				Floranthe
			Fanny Dawon	Nabocklish
				Miss Tooley
		Pocahontas	Glencoe	Sultan
				Trampoline
			Marpessa	Muley
				Clare
	Adeline	Ion	Cain	Paulowitz
				Daughter Of Paynator
			Margaret	Edmund
				Medora
		Little Fairy	Hornsea	----------------

			Lacerta	Zodiac
				Jerboa

Best progenitor of the Pocahontas heart line through his daughters

Storm Cat
1983

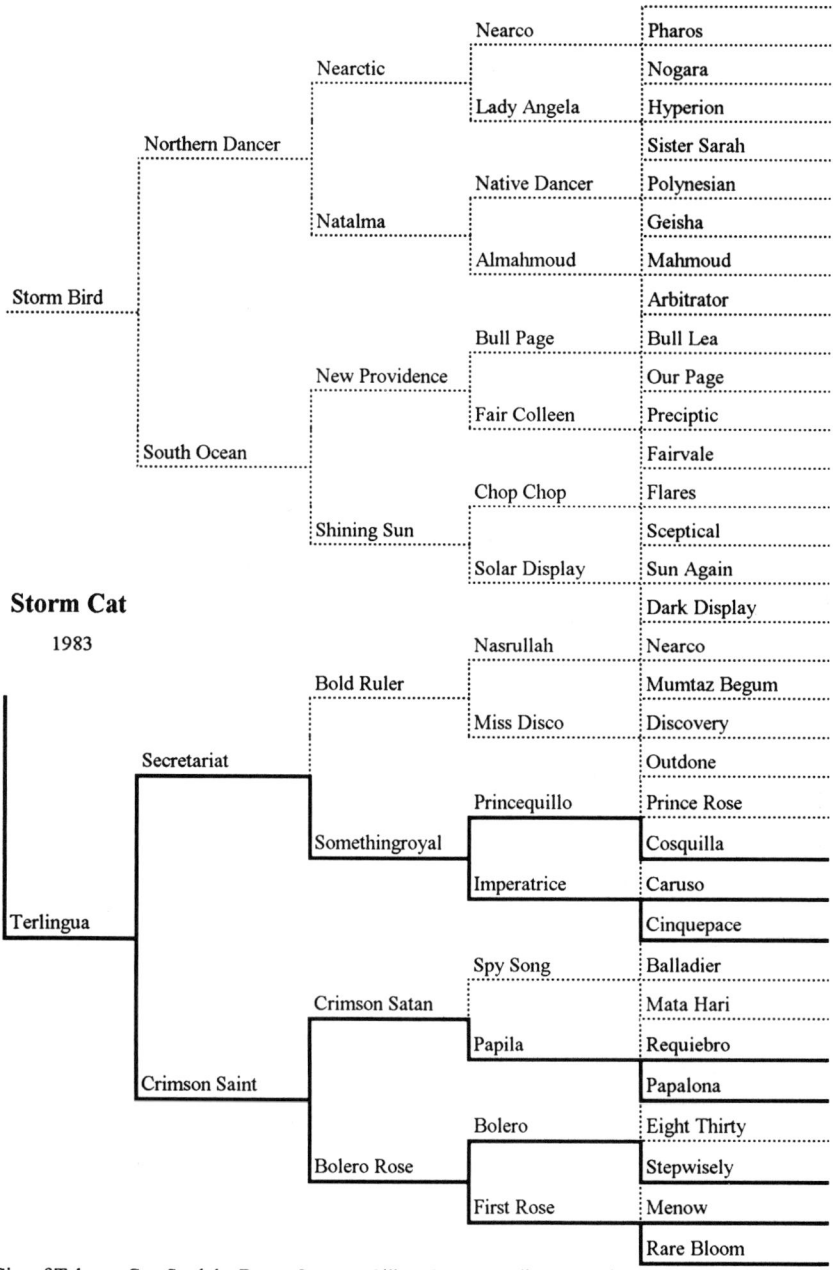

Pedigree:

- Storm Bird
  - Northern Dancer
    - Nearctic
      - Nearco
        - Pharos
        - Nogara
      - Lady Angela
        - Hyperion
        - Sister Sarah
    - Natalma
      - Native Dancer
        - Polynesian
        - Geisha
      - Almahmoud
        - Mahmoud
        - Arbitrator
  - South Ocean
    - New Providence
      - Bull Page
        - Bull Lea
        - Our Page
      - Fair Colleen
        - Preciptic
        - Fairvale
    - Shining Sun
      - Chop Chop
        - Flares
        - Sceptical
      - Solar Display
        - Sun Again
        - Dark Display

- Terlingua
  - Secretariat
    - Bold Ruler
      - Nasrullah
        - Nearco
        - Mumtaz Begum
      - Miss Disco
        - Discovery
        - Outdone
    - Somethingroyal
      - Princequillo
        - Prince Rose
        - Cosquilla
      - Imperatrice
        - Caruso
        - Cinquepace
  - Crimson Saint
    - Crimson Satan
      - Spy Song
        - Balladier
        - Mata Hari
      - Papila
        - Requiebro
        - Papalona
    - Bolero Rose
      - Bolero
        - Eight Thirty
        - Stepwisely
      - First Rose
        - Menow
        - Rare Bloom

Sire of Tabasco Cat, Sardula, Desert Stormer, Silken Cat - Canadian champion

Swaps
1952

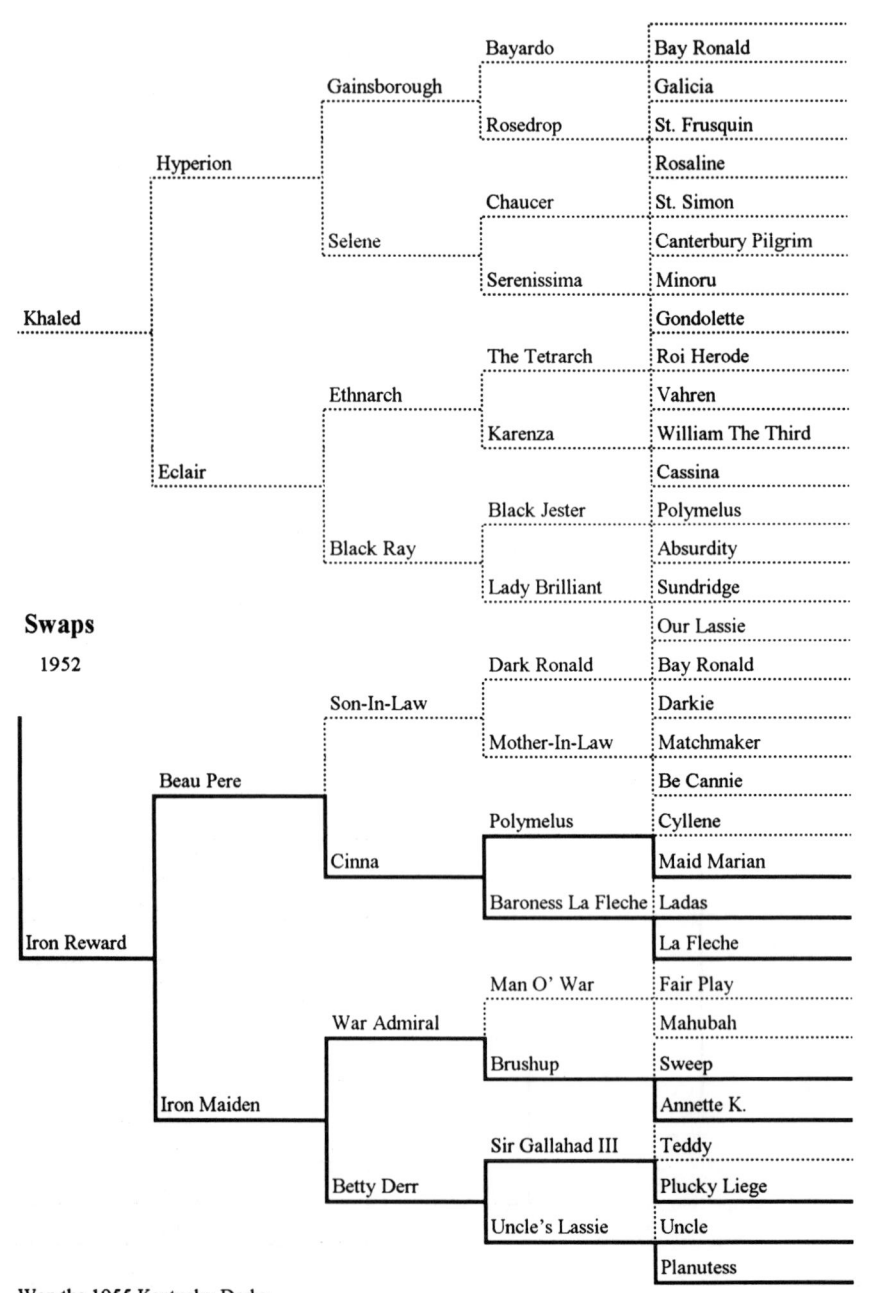

Khaled
- Hyperion
  - Gainsborough
    - Bayardo
      - Bay Ronald
      - Galicia
    - Rosedrop
      - St. Frusquin
      - Rosaline
  - Selene
    - Chaucer
      - St. Simon
      - Canterbury Pilgrim
    - Serenissima
      - Minoru
      - Gondolette
- Eclair
  - Ethnarch
    - The Tetrarch
      - Roi Herode
      - Vahren
    - Karenza
      - William The Third
      - Cassina
  - Black Ray
    - Black Jester
      - Polymelus
      - Absurdity
    - Lady Brilliant
      - Sundridge
      - Our Lassie

Iron Reward
- Beau Pere
  - Son-In-Law
    - Dark Ronald
      - Bay Ronald
      - Darkie
    - Mother-In-Law
      - Matchmaker
      - Be Cannie
  - Cinna
    - Polymelus
      - Cyllene
      - Maid Marian
    - Baroness La Fleche
      - Ladas
      - La Fleche
- Iron Maiden
  - War Admiral
    - Man O' War
      - Fair Play
      - Mahubah
    - Brushup
      - Sweep
      - Annette K.
  - Betty Derr
    - Sir Gallahad III
      - Teddy
      - Plucky Liege
    - Uncle's Lassie
      - Uncle
      - Planutess

Won the 1955 Kentucky Derby

Tracery
1909

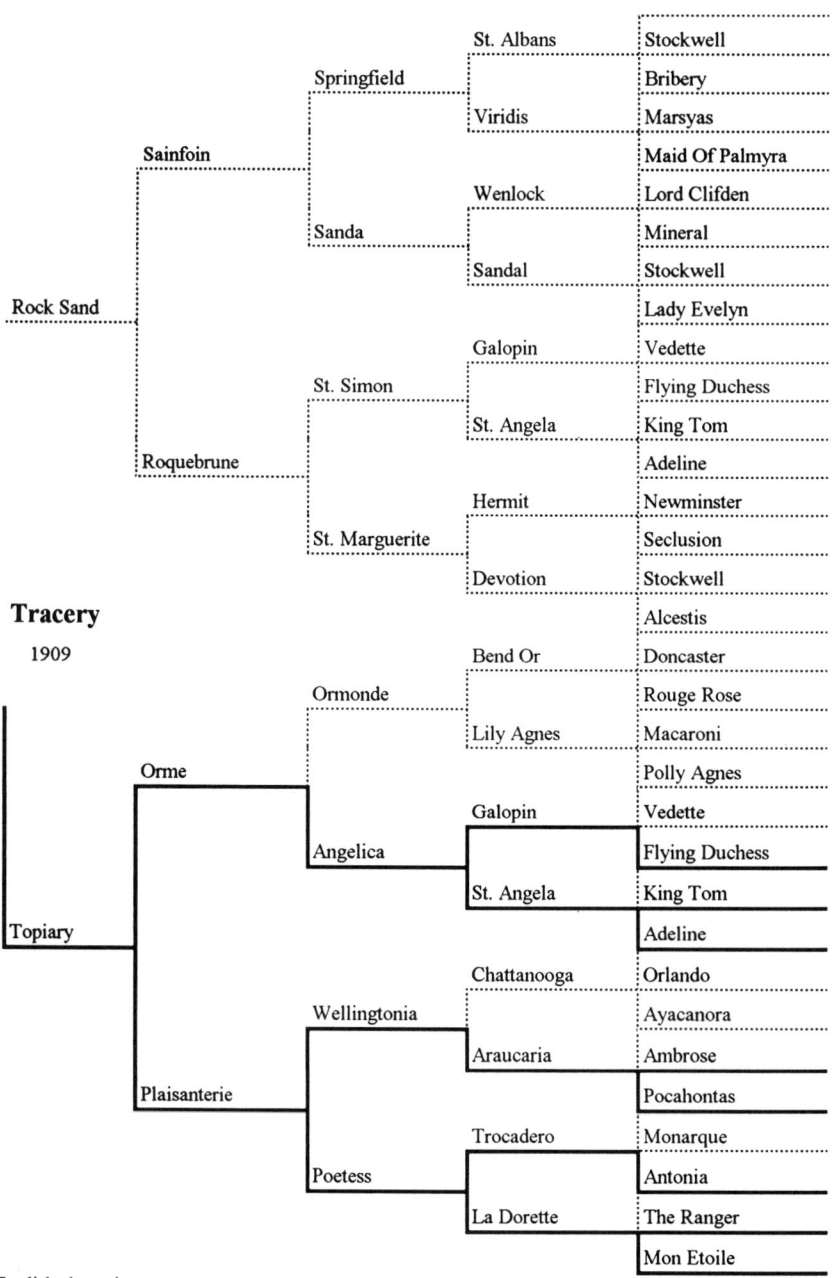

Rock Sand	Sainfoin	Springfield	St. Albans	Stockwell
				Bribery
			Viridis	Marsyas
				Maid Of Palmyra
		Sanda	Wenlock	Lord Clifden
				Mineral
			Sandal	Stockwell
				Lady Evelyn
	Roquebrune	St. Simon	Galopin	Vedette
				Flying Duchess
			St. Angela	King Tom
				Adeline
		St. Marguerite	Hermit	Newminster
				Seclusion
			Devotion	Stockwell
				Alcestis
Topiary	Orme	Ormonde	Bend Or	Doncaster
				Rouge Rose
			Lily Agnes	Macaroni
				Polly Agnes
		Angelica	Galopin	Vedette
				Flying Duchess
			St. Angela	King Tom
				Adeline
	Plaisanterie	Wellingtonia	Chattanooga	Orlando
				Ayacanora
			Araucaria	Ambrose
				Pocahontas
		Poetess	Trocadero	Monarque
				Antonia
			La Dorette	The Ranger
				Mon Etoile

English champion
Winner of St. Leger
Sire of Teresina and Papyrus - winner of the English Derby

197

Index

A.P. Assay, 104
A.P. Indy, 75, 77, 87-88, 104-105, 109, 145, 168
Academy Award, 114
Ack Ack, 109
Admiral Drake, 143, 147
Adored, 81
Affirmed, 75, 114
Afleet, 109, 129
Air Forbes One, 129
Ajax, 141
Al Mamoon, 109
Alablue, 114, 118
Albatross, 49
Alcibiades, 89
Alibhai, 104, 141, 143
All Rainbows, 59
Alleged, 75, 117, 119
Allen's Prospect, 114
Alluvial, 79, 89
Almahmoud, 89, 122, 147
Althea, 38, 89, 163-164
Always Mint, 105
Alydar, 75, 117-119, 163
Alydeed, 117, 119
Alysheba, 75, 114
Andromaque, 112
Apremont, 68
Araucaria, 68, 89, 141
Arazi, 122-123
Arnie Almahurst, 47
Arrazi, 75
Aspidistra, 89, 113
Aunt Hilda, 53
Auraria, 68
Aurum, 68
Baby League, 89, 112
Ball Belle, 47
Ballerina Gal, 108
Baltic Speed, 51
Banish Fear, 118, 147, 152
Barbicue Sauce, 105
Bates Motel, 117, 119
Bathing Girl, 89
Batonnier, 117, 119
Be Faithful, 89, 119
Beaming Beauty, 112
Beau Pere, 163
Becker, 109
Bee Mac, 89, 113
Bel Sheba, 89
Believe It, 75, 114
Belthazar, 89
Ben Brush, 137
Bend Or, 141
Bergsten, G., 47
Bet Twice, 111, 114, 130
Better Self, 113-114
Betty's Secret, 89

Betty Derr, 164
Bewitch, 53
Big Spruce, 117, 119
Bimlette, 119
Bird Flower, 89
Black Helen, 89
Black Servant, 117-118
Black Tie Affair, 75
Blenheim II, 121
Bloodroot, 89, 119, 163
Blossom Time, 117-118
Blue Banner, 89-90, 101, 118
Blue Delight, 118
Blue Denim, 89, 118
Blue Grass, 149
Blue Hen, 165
Blue Larkspur, 75, 79, 83, 95, 101, 112, 114, 117-119, 143, 147, 152-153, 163-164
Blue Swords, 104
Blushing Groom, 103
Blushing John, 117, 119
Boat, 89
body type, 89, 91, 94, 105, 143-144, 169
Bois Roussel, 143
Bold Bidder, 109
Bold Hour, 59
Bold Reason, 117, 119
Bold Ruler, 23, 42, 70-71, 137, 139, 141, 170, 174
Boldnesian, 117-119
Bornastar, 143
Bosra Sham, 112
Boudoir II, 89
Bowl Of Flowers, 143
Bramalea, 89
Break Through, 104
Bright Beam, 73
Bright Candles, 112
Broad Brush, 114
Broadway, 89
broodmare sire, 49, 53, 74, 77, 79, 85, 87, 89, 95, 111, 113, 118, 122, 128-129, 139, 141, 144, 147, 152, 167-168
Brush Up, 111-112
Brushup, 89, 139
Bubbling Over, 112, 137
Buckpasser, 75, 79, 83, 87, 103, 112-114, 118-119, 143-145, 153, 163-164, 171
Bull Dog, 143
Bull Lea, 145
Bull Page, 118
Bupers, 114

Busanda, 75, 79, 89, 103, 112, 118, 153, 164
Busher, 75, 79, 89, 104, 112
Businesslike, 89, 112, 118, 153
But Why Not, 75
Byars, Dr. Doug, 158
Cahill Road, 113-114
Camel, 65
Canterbury Pilgrimage, 144
Cap and Bells, 89
Capote, 75
cardiac output, 19, 28, 30, 40-41, 47, 69-70, 149
Caress, 105
Caro, 23, 42, 59, 70, 73
Carry The Message, 47
Castleton Farm, 47
Cat Appeal, 105
Cat Attack, 105
Caveat, 117, 119
Cequillo, 113
Challedon, 75, 143
Chanzi, 112
Chapel of Dreams, 89
Chaucer, 141, 144
Check Off Dollars, 125-126
Cheery Hello, 49
Chenery, Christopher, 170
Chenery, Penny, 18, 71, 91, 169-176
Cherokee Run, 107
Chester, 68
Chief's Crown, 75, 109
Chiola Hanover, 49
Choral Group, 129
Cigar, 79, 81, 112, 141
Citation, 75, 129, 152, 167
Clandestina, 81, 83, 128
Cohoes, 117, 119
Coined Silver, 129
Con Game, 89
Concertina, 143
conformation, 23, 27, 70, 89, 91, 93
Continentalvictory, 49, 53, 168
Corporate Report, 109
Corrazona, 112
Cosmah, 89, 147
Cosmic Bomb, 118, 147
Cosquilla, 89, 92, 99
Costill, David L., 19-20
Cothran, Gus, 25, 65-69, 94, 164-165
Cougar II, 175

Count Fleet, 75, 143
Country Cat, 105
Courtly Dee, 89, 163-164
Cozzene, 75, 152
Crafty Admiral, 75, 114
Crimson Saint, 89
Crimson Satan, 75
Croll, Jimmy, 149, 151
Cryptoclearance, 114
Crystal Gazing, 112
Cunningham, 62
Cure The Blues, 75, 114
Damascus, 75, 117, 119
Danzig, 75
Danzig Connection, 109
Dark Lomond, 81
Dayjur, 117, 119
Dearly Precious, 113
Defensive Play, 109
Dehere, 75, 105, 109, 168
DeMar, Clarence, 20
DeMaria, Dr. Anthony, 159
Demons' Begone, 122-123
Desert Gold, 68
Desert Secret, 38, 81, 83, 103, 114, 128-129, 141
Desert Stormer, 105
Devil's Bag, 75, 117, 119
Devotion, 141
Dinner Time, 143
Diplomat Way, 79, 109
Discovery, 137
distance runners, 19
Dixie Brass, 109
DNA, 68-69, 94, 164
Dominant Dancer, 108
Donatella III, 122
Doncaster, 122
dosage system, 24-25
double copy, 62, 67, 85, 87, 89, 101, 111, 113, 128, 144-145, 153, 163, 165, 168
Double Jay, 87
Dr. Blum, 109
Dr. Fager, 75, 113-114, 141
Dustwhirl, 111-112
Easy Goer, 38, 75, 113-114, 163-164
ECG, 19, 28-31, 43-44, 68-69, 123, 144-145, 151, 153, 155-158
echocardiography, 158, 160
Eclipse, 27, 38, 65, 67-68, 71, 73-75, 95, 133, 143
Educated Risk, 103
Eight Thirty, 143

198

El Gran Senor, 75, 112, 114, 141
electrocardiogram, 28-29, 69, 151
Elpis, 118
Elrafa Ah, 105
Emily's Pride, 49, 53
Entropy, 113
Everlasting, 67
Express Ride, 47
Fair Charmer, 79, 119
Fall Aspen, 89
Fappiano, 75, 113-114
Fariman, 118
Farma Way, 109
Fast Gold, 109
Fast Play, 114
Ferdinand, 75
First Flight, 122
Fit To Fight, 103
Flaming Page, 89, 118, 129
Flaming Swords, 104
Flaming Top, 129
Flanders, 112
Flitabout, 89
Florican, 47
Flory Messenger, 47, 51, 53
Flower Bowl, 89, 104, 143
Flowing, 112
Flutter Away, 81
Fly So Free, 117, 119
Flying Continental, 122-123
For My Mom, 108
Fort Marcy, 75, 101, 103, 118
Forty Niner, 75, 109
Fractious, 67
Fraxinella, 67
Fregin, Dr. Frederick, 41, 68-69, 151, 155-158
Full Pocket, 129
Gaga, 89
Gainsborough, 121, 141
Gale Force, 104
Galla Colors, 147
Gallant Man, 122-123
Gallorette, 75
Gana Facil, 89, 113
Gay Gallanta, 112
Gay Matelda, 170
Gay Missle, 89
Geisha, 137
General Assembly, 104, 168
genetic marker, 68-69, 145, 164
genetic mutation, 65, 71
genetics, 25-26, 28, 57, 94
Genovefa, 112
Glencoe, 67
Glorious Song, 89

Go Step, 118
Gold Digger, 119
Golden Opinion, 79
Gone West, 75, 109, 168
Gorgeous, 79
Graustark, 122-123, 143
Great Above, 113-114
Green Dancer, 117, 119
Grey Dawn II, 119, 122-123
Grey Flight, 122
greyhound, 20, 33, 40
Hail To Reason, 104, 147
Halo, 75, 118-119, 122-123, 147, 152
Hancock, A.B., 172
Hancock, Seth, 171-172
heart line, 49, 51, 53, 59, 68, 71, 79, 81, 83, 89, 95, 101, 107, 111, 113-114, 126, 129, 133, 137, 141, 143- 145, 147, 152, 155, 162, 164, 166
heart score, 16, 23, 28-31, 33-45, 47, 49, 51, 53, 57, 59, 61-62, 68-70, 73, 81, 83, 95, 99, 103, 105, 108, 123, 125, 128, 133, 145, 151-153, 155
heart weight, 20, 28, 37-41, 47, 69
Heavenly Prize, 112
heterozygous, 165
Higdon, Hal, 20
His Majesty, 104, 122-123
Hoist The Flag, 113-114
Holy Bull, 75, 122-123, 149
Homebuilder, 122-123
homozygous, 62, 87, 128, 165
Hopespringseternal, 89, 145
Housebuster, 114
Hum Along, 113
Hunter Genetics, 93
Hyperion, 38, 122, 129, 144
Iberia, 170
Imperatrice, 89-90, 169
Inchmurrin, 81
inheritance, 28, 57, 59, 61-62, 68-69, 128
Inside Information, 103
Instep, 68
intelligence, 93-94
Intercontinental, 53
Irish Open, 114
Isinglas, 141
Isonomy, 141
Ivatan, 129
Ivy Road, 152

Jet Action, 79, 112
Jewell Princess, 103
Jewell Ridge, 103
John Henry, 75, 87
John O'Gaunt, 141
Jones, William E., 24
Joy Baby, 105
Judy-Rae, 163
Karen's Choice, 51
Kathie's Colleen, 112
Kaufman, Dr. Walter, 13
Kelso, 75
Kerala, 89
Key Bridge, 89-91, 99, 101, 103, 118
Key Contender, 103, 109
Key To Content, 118
Key To The Kingdom, 75, 103, 118
Key To The Mint, 16, 38, 75, 93, 99, 101, 103, 105, 109, 118, 152, 157, 175
Key Witness, 103
Keystone Starlet, 53
Killaloe, 38, 89, 113
King Tom, 68, 141, 143
Kingston Town, 38
Kris S, 75, 109
L'Alezane, 113
La Chica, 104
La Troienne, 89
Lady Angela, 89
Lady Chester, 68
Lady Josephine, 89
Lady Lark, 118
Lady's Secret, 75, 104
Lakeway, 81
Lambert, Dr. David, 159-160
Landaluce, 81
Lassie Dear, 87, 92, 144-145
Laurin, Lucien, 170, 172
Le Slew, 81
Leading Ballerina, 108
Letalong, 51
Life At The Top, 81
Light Lark, 118
Lindy Lane, 168
Little Missouri, 117, 119
Lomond, 81, 114
Look Up, 143
Lord Durham, 129
Lucratif, 114
Mack Lobell, 51
Mackie, 104
Mah Mahal, 89, 121
Mahmoud, 75, 83, 95, 121-123, 145, 147, 149
Majestic Prince, 122-123
Majideh, 122
Malachite, 143
Malleret, 104

Man O' War, 75, 95, 105, 111, 139, 141, 143, 173
Manikato, 38
Maplejinsky, 89
Marling, 81
Marpessa, 67
Masaka, 122
Medaille D'Or, 168
Melyno, 103
Memories Of Donny, 105
Mendal, 94
Menow, 75
Mesabi, 152
Metfield, 129
Mickey McGuire, 122-123
Milan Mill, 74, 89, 91, 105
Mill Reef, 27, 38, 40, 73-75, 93, 105, 109, 114, 123
Millicent, 89, 105
Mining, 114
Miss Carmie, 59, 89
Miss Disco, 139
Miss Dogwood, 119
Miss Zigby, 89
Missed The Storm, 105
Misty Morn, 75, 89, 122
Miswaki, 75, 145
Mocassin, 75, 89
Mochila, 152
Mock Orange, 113
Momote, 29
Morgan, Dr. Thomas Hunt, 94
Moscow Ballet, 30, 38, 91, 93, 105, 107-109, 123, 125, 128
Moscow TV, 108
Most Happy Fella, 49
Mountain Cat, 105, 109, 152
Movin' Money, 152
Mr. Prospector, 117, 119
Mr. Thrifty, 123
Mumtaz Begum, 89
Mumtaz Mahal, 89, 121-122
My Charmer, 79, 81, 89, 103, 112, 119, 128
My Dear Girl, 75, 89
My Flag, 112
Myrtle Charm, 75, 119
Myrtlewood, 75, 89, 119
Nadean, 68
Nashua, 75
Nasrullah, 121-122, 145
Natalma, 89, 122
Native Dancer, 75, 104, 137, 139
Naval Orange, 89, 113
Navarra, 112
Never Bend, 74, 163

Nielsen and Vibe-
    Petersen, 34-36, 43-45,
    47
Night Shift, 75, 159
Nijinsky II, 74-75, 81,
    117-119, 129
Noble Lassie, 89
Noble Victory, 49, 53
North Star III, 118
Northern Dancer, 38, 75,
    81, 122-123, 159
Nothirdchance, 104, 147
November Snow, 105
Numbered Account, 89
Nureyev, 75
Nurmi, Paavo, 20
Ocean Cat, 105
Ogygian, 75
Omaha, 75, 129, 167
One For All, 109
Onion, 175
OP Cat, 105
Opening Verse, 122-123
Orbit's Scene, 129
Our Page, 118
Padilla, 118
Pancho Villa, 168
Peace Corps, 51, 53
Personal Ensign, 89, 112
Personal Flag, 114
Personal Hope, 117, 119
Pert Flirt, 49
Phalaris, 141
Phar Lap, 17, 38, 68
Phipps, Ogden, 71
Piccalili, 129
Pine Bluff, 122-123
Pink Domino, 111, 137
Playmate, 152
Pleasant Colony, 75, 109
Plucky Liege, 89, 143,
    147
Plugged Nickle, 114
Pocahontas, 24, 65, 67-68,
    71, 75, 77, 87, 95, 104-
    105, 111, 129, 133,
    137, 141, 143-145, 147,
    164
Poker, 79, 112
Polish Navy, 75
Portage, 152
Prayer Bell, 89
Prince Courtauld, 28-29
Prince John, 117-119, 152
Prince Rose, 92, 99
Princequillo, 31, 65, 71,
    73-75, 79, 83, 89-93,
    95, 99, 101, 103, 105,
    107, 109, 113, 118,
    125, 144-145, 152
Private Account, 75, 103,
    112, 114, 141
Proud Truth, 129
Pure Profit, 103

QRS complex, 19, 29-30,
    151
Quack, 109
Quebracho, 73
Quick Cure, 114
Quickly, 89, 143
Quiet American, 114
Quill, 75
Rahy, 75, 122-123
Rainbows For Life, 122-
    123
Ran-Tan, 129
Rantanen, Norman, 94,
    151, 158-160
Rare Mint, 89
Rare Performer, 114
Rataplan, 68, 141
Real Delight, 118
Red Ransom, 117, 119
regression coefficients,
    59, 61-62
Relaunch, 117, 119
Relaxing, 89
Ribbon, 104
Ride The Trails, 152
Risen Star, 104, 122-123,
    168
Risque, 101
Risque Blue, 101, 118
Riva Ridge, 170, 175
Riverman, 117, 119
Roberto, 117, 119
Robin Des Pins, 109
Rock Sand, 141, 143
Roi Herod, 141
Roman, 143
Romanella, 89
Roquebrune, 141
Rough Shod II, 89
Royal Prestige, 47
Sadler's Wells, 75, 83
Sadler's Wells, 81
Sainfoin, 141
Sandal, 68
Sardula, 105
Sauce Boat, 105
Seaplane, 143
Seattle Dancer, 81
Seattle Meteor, 81
Seattle Slew, 75, 77, 79,
    81, 88, 103, 108, 112,
    114, 119, 128, 141
Secretame, 89
Secretariat, 11-13, 17-18,
    26-27, 31, 38, 40, 59,
    62, 65, 70-71, 75, 77,
    81, 85, 87, 91-93, 103-
    105, 109, 128, 137,
    143-144, 163, 168-176
Seeking The Gold, 75,
    103, 112, 114, 141
Selene, 89, 144
Senate Appointee, 105
Sequence, 89, 119

sex linkage, 57, 65, 93-94,
    166
Sexy Slew, 79
Sham, 13, 17, 27, 31, 38,
    40, 65, 103, 109, 163
Sharon Brown, 89
Shayne McGuire, 123
Sherzarcat, 105
Shy Dawn, 89
Silent Screen, 75, 114
Silken Cat, 105
Silver Ghost, 122-123
Silver Spoon, 129
Sir Gallahad III, 75, 105,
    143, 147, 164
Sir Gaylord, 109, 144,
    152, 170
Sir Harry Lewis, 122-123
Sissy's Time, 125, 128
Sister Dot, 105
Six Crowns, 89
Skip Away, 79
Skip Trial, 122-123
Sky Classic, 75
Skywalker, 117, 119
Slew City Slew, 109
Slew O' Gold, 79
Slewacide, 129
Slewpy, 117, 119
smart genes, 94
Smile, 117, 119
Solar Slew, 79, 81, 89,
    112
Somethingfabulous, 109
Somethingroyal, 71, 89-
    91, 137, 145, 152, 169-
    170
Source Sucree, 147
South Ocean, 89
Sovereign Dancer, 122-
    123
Soviet Problem, 38, 107-
    108, 156
Special, 89
Spectacular Bid, 75, 122-
    123
St. Angela, 141, 143
St. Simon, 141, 143
Stage Flite, 129
stakes earnings, 45
Stalwart, 117, 119
Standardbred, 168
Standardbreds, 34-36, 61,
    70, 151
Star's Pride, 47, 49, 53
Star Kingdom, 27, 38
State Dinner, 122-123
Steel, Dr. James D., 28-
    29, 31, 33, 36-37, 39-
    42, 44, 47, 61, 69-70,
    151, 155
Stellar Cat, 105
Stewart, Dr. Anthony, 23,
    33-37, 40-42, 44, 57,
    59, 61-62, 69-70, 73,
    151, 155
Stockwell, 68, 137, 141
Stop The Music, 172
Storm Bird, 75, 88
Storm Cat, 75, 105, 109,
    168
Storm Song, 104, 113
Strategic Maneuver, 114
Strike a Balance, 89
Striking, 79, 89, 112
stroke volume, 28, 30, 41,
    47, 69
Successor, 109
Sugar Squeeze, 104
Summer Squall, 77, 87-
    88, 104-105, 109, 113,
    145, 168
Summer Tan, 129
Sundridge, 141
Super Bowl, 47, 53
Swaps, 75, 114
Sweep, 104, 111-112,
    114, 129, 137, 139,
    143-144
Sweep On, 139
Sweeping Glance, 143
Sweet Lavender, 147
Sweet Tooth, 89, 118
Swerczek, Dr. Thomas,
    12-13, 17, 26, 59, 163
Sword Dance, 109
Swynford, 147
Syrian Sea, 170
T.V. Lark, 117-119
Ta Wee, 113
Tabasco Cat, 105
Tactile, 79
Tamerett, 89
Tar Heel, 51
Tarport Cheer, 49, 51
Tarport Hap, 49
Tasso, 122-123
Teleran, 89
Tempest Dancer, 105
Teresa Mc, 108, 123
Terlingua, 89, 105
The Last Red, 38, 91,
    125-126, 128
The Meadow, 169-170
Timeform, 34-35
Toll Booth, 89
Tom Fool, 75
Tom Rolfe, 75, 109
Top Knight, 129
Topiary, 141
Toussaud, 112
Tracery, 104, 141
Tulle, 163
Tulloch, 38
Tulyar, 74
Turner, GIllian, 93-94
Turn-To, 147
Twilight Tear, 118
Tyler B, 49

200

Ultimus, 143
ultrasound, 62, 94, 125, 144-145, 149, 151, 158, 160, 162
Unbridled, 75, 113-114
University of Sydney, 28
Vaguely Noble, 75
Vaila, 118
Valley Victory, 49, 51, 53, 168
Via Borghese, 81
Vo Rogue, 38
Volomite, 51, 53
Vuillier, Colonel, 24
Waquoit, 122-123

War Admiral, 75, 79, 81, 83, 95, 101, 103-104, 111-114, 118, 128-129, 137, 139, 141, 143-144, 152-153, 163-164
Wavering Monarch, 114
Wavy Navy, 89, 113
Weekend Surprise, 77, 87-88, 92-93, 104-105, 144-145
Wellingtonia, 141
Welsh Pageant, 73-74
What A Pleasure, 122-123
Whirla Lea, 130

Whirlaway, 75, 111, 114, 129-130, 135, 137, 167
White, Henry, 25
Whitney, C. V., 122
Winning Color, 59
Winning Colors, 59
With Approval, 70, 75, 114, 141
Wolfhound, 145
Won't Tell You, 89
Wood Of Binn, 112
Woodbine, 104, 137
Woodman, 75, 112, 114, 141, 152
Woodpecker, 67

Worth Beein', 53
X chromosome, 20, 25, 31, 35, 47, 57, 59, 62, 65, 68-69, 71, 75, 77, 79, 85, 87, 89, 93-95, 111-113, 128, 133, 135, 139, 143-145, 153, 155, 163, 165-168
X-Factor, 68, 71, 75, 139, 163
You'd Be Surprised, 103
Zanthe, 117, 119

Names in Pedigrees

Abbedale, 50
Abbots Anne, 186
Abbots Trace, 186-187
Abernant, 150
Absurdity, 196
Abyssinia II, 150
Adeline, 142, 191, 194, 197
Adioo, 50
Adioo Guy, 50
Adioo Volo, 50
Adios, 50
Admiral Drake, 146
Adriana, 134, 136
Adrienne, 14, 134, 136
Advocate, 187
Aerolite, 110, 140
Affection, 78
Agathea, 150
Agathea's Dawn, 150
Agneta, 116
Ajax, 154, 179-180-183, 188, 191-192
Al Hattab, 150
Alablue, 76, 78, 193
Alanesian, 76, 78, 193
Alarm, 138
Albia, 110, 127, 138
Alcestis, 142, 197
Alcibiades, 78, 86, 106, 180, 184, 190
Ale, 150
Alexander, 66
Alexander mare, 66
Alibhai, 100, 124
Alice, 191
All Rainbows, 58
Allemande, 184
Allie Song, 46
Alluvial, 78
Almahmoud, 82, 106, 124, 146, 186-187, 193, 195
Aloe, 80
Alpoise, 78, 86, 180, 184, 190
Alsab, 76, 78, 80, 82
Althea, 178
Alxanth, 150
Alydar, 178-179, 184
Amazon, 66
Ambitious Blaze, 46
Ambrose, 197
American Flag, 178-179, 184, 190
Americus, 120
Americus Girl, 120, 134
Amie, 154, 182, 181, 188
Amphion, 116, 120, 188
Ampola, 150, 185
Anchora, 134, 186
Angelic, 116, 154, 181
Angelica, 191, 197

Annette K., 100, 102, 110, 154, 178, 180-181, 196
Anomaly, 127
Antonia, 197
Apelle, 100
Appleby, 185
Araucaria, 197
Arbitrator, 82, 106, 146, 186-187, 195
Arctic Night, 58
Arethusa, 66
Argot Hal, 50
Ariadne, 14, 86, 134, 136, 179, 186
Aristophanes, 82, 187
Armenia, 188
Arnie, 191
Arnie Almahurst, 46
Aspidistra, 150, 183
Assignation, 14, 86, 192
Asta, 191
Asterus, 72
Atalanta, 188
Audience, 136
Aunt Hilda, 52
Australian, 110, 138, 140
Ayacanora, 197
Ayn Hali, 80
Ayrshire, 120, 127, 188
Baba Kenny, 183
Baby League, 76, 80, 181
Bacchante, 66
Ball Belle, 46
Balladier, 58, 195
Ballot, 182
Baltic Speed, 48, 52
Banish Fear, 146, 189
Bar The Way, 98, 102, 189, 192
Barbara Burrini, 100
Barbelle, 194
Baroness La Fleche, 196
Barrier, 14, 72, 98, 100, 102, 189, 192
Barrisdale, 98
Bathing Girl, 102, 110, 154, 180-181
Baton Rouge, 146
Batter Up, 193
Bay Flower, 138
Bay Leaf, 138
Bay Middleton, 194
Bay Ronald, 98, 120, 154, 181-182, 188, 191, 196
Bayardo, 98, 102, 120, 182, 185-186, 189, 192, 196
Bayou, 78
Baytown, 58
Be Cannie, 196
Be Faithful, 72, 82, 178
Beaming Beauty, 181
Beau Pere, 100, 178, 196

Beaudesert, 110, 127, 138
Bee Mac, 150, 183
Beeswing, 142
Bel Agnes, 185
Belgravia, 116, 154, 183
Bella Fia, 193
Bella Minna, 100
Belle Rose, 110, 127, 138, 154, 181
Bellini, 100
Bellinzona, 116
Bellisario, 181
Beloved, 178-179, 184, 190
Ben Brush, 102, 110, 116, 127, 136, 138, 154, 180-181
Ben Holiday, 127
Bend Or, 110, 116, 127, 140, 154, 181, 188, 191, 197
Bendigo, 120, 127
Beningbrough, 66
Beppo, 98, 185
Berkshire Chimes, 50
Berriedale, 127
Bert Abbe, 50
Better Self, 150, 183
Betty Beall, 183
Betty Crispin, 50
Betty Derr, 178, 196
Betty G., 50
Beverly Hanover, 46
Bewitch, 52
Bexley, 52
Big Event, 150
Big Game, 150
Big Hurry, 184
Bill And Coo, 179
Bill Gallon, 46, 48
Billy Direct, 50
Bimelech, 72, 150, 178, 183
Bingen, 50
Bird Flower, 190
Bird Loose, 136
Birdcatcher, 194
Biturica, 181
Bizerte, 193
Black Cherry, 120, 127
Black Corrie, 191
Black Curl, 80
Black Duchess, 120, 127, 191
Black Helen, 124
Black Jester, 196
Black Maria, 136
Black Polly, 76, 124, 136, 178-179, 184, 186-187, 190
Black Queen, 136, 179, 186
Black Ray, 72, 196

Black Servant, 100, 102, 116, 146, 154, 180, 183, 185, 189
Black Toney, 72, 102, 116, 136, 154, 180, 183-184, 189
Black Wave, 76, 80
Blackball, 150
Blacklock, 194
Blair Athol, 138
Blanche, 120, 127, 134, 185
Blandford, 14, 72, 80, 120, 127, 134, 146, 185-187
Blaze Hanover, 46
Blenheim II, 14, 72, 76, 80, 86, 120, 127, 134, 146, 150, 178-179, 185-187
Blessings, 179
Bloodroot, 72, 178
Blossom Time, 100, 102, 116, 146, 154, 180, 185, 189
Blue Banner, 100, 102
Blue Delight, 178-179, 184
Blue Denim, 185
Blue Glass, 186
Blue Grass, 136, 179
Blue Larkspur, 72, 76, 78, 80, 86, 100, 102, 106, **116,** 146, 154, 179-180, 184-185, 189-190
Blue Rose, 127
Blue Swords, 76, 146
Blue Tit, 100
Boat, 124
Bold Hitter, 193
Bold Hour, 58
Bold Reason, 82
Bold Reasoning, 76, 78
Bold Ruler, 14, 58, 76, 78, 82, 86, 106, 124, **134,** 193, 195
Boldnesian, 76, 78, 193
Bolero, 195
Bolero Rose, 195
Bona Vista, 120
Bonefish, 48
Bonnie Doon, 116
Bonnie Scotland, 110, 127, 138
Bonny Gal, 116
Bosworth, 185
Boudoir II, 100, 124
Bourtai, 78
Boxeuse, 185
Bramble, 110, 116, 127, 138, 154, 181
Breathless, 150

202

Brenda Hanover, 52
Bribery, 142, 197
Bridal Colors, 58
Bridge Of Sighs, 134, 136
Brielle, 192
Broad Corrie, 182
Broad Ripple, 187
Broadway, 190
Brocatelle, 80
Brokers Tip, 184
Bromus, 134, 136, 146, 180, 186
Broomielaw, 140
Broomstick, 136
Brown Bread, 140
Brown Bud, 14, 86, 192
Brown Prince, 14, 192
Brownhylda, 185
Brushup, 78, 80, 86, 100, 102, 110, 154, 178, 180-181, 183-184, 190, 196
Bubbling Over, 78, 80, 181
Buckpasser, 78, 86, **180**, 184, 190
Buckup, 190
Bucolic, 100
Bull Brier, 150, 183
Bull Dog, 78, 86, 106, 150, 179-180, 182-184, 190
Bull Lea, 58, 106, 124, 178-179, 182, 184, 193-195
Bull Page, 106, 124, 193, 195
Burgoo King, 124
Busanda, 78, 86, **154**, 180, 184, 190
Busher, 76, 78, 80, 82, **181**
Businesslike, 78, 86, 154, 180, 184, 190
Buzz Fuzz, 150
Buzzard, 66
Cain, 194
Calash, 66
Callistrate, 98
Calumet Aristocrat, 46
Calumet Chuck, 48
Cameronian, 58
Canterbury Pilgrim, 110, 120, 127, 154, 181-182, 196
Carbine, 110, 182, 188, 191
Carlisle, 48, 52
Caro, 58
Carolyn, 46
Caruso, 14, 82, 86, 106, 192, 195
Case Ace, 178-179, 184-185, 190
Cassina, 196

Castania, 120
Catnip, 14, 72, 134, 186-187
Cavaliere d'Arpino, 100
Celt, 188
Cerito, 182
Challedon, 190
Challenger II, 190
Chambord, 58
Chamossaire, 58
Chance Shot, 146, 186
Charles O'Malley, 120, 127, 134, 185
Chattanooga, 197
Chaucer, 134, 136, 146, 180, 182, 186, 196
Chelandry, 188
Chicle, 146, 183, 186
Chicleight, 179
Chiola Hanover, 48
Chop Chop, 195
Cicuta, 14, 134, 136
Cinderella, 110, 116, 140, 154, 181
Cinna, 100, 178, 196
Cinq A Sept, 14, 192
Cinquepace, 14, 82, 86, 106, 192, 195
Cita Frisco, 50
Citation, **182**
Clamart, 191
Clandestina, 82
Clang, 58
Clare, 66, 194
Clemence, 191
Cleopatra, 14, 134, 136, 180
Cloak, 134
Clorinda Hanover, 48
Clorita Hanover, 48
Clotilde Hanover, 48
Cobweb, 194
Colonel Armstrong, 50
Colonial, 182
Comic Song, 182, 188, 191
Commando, 116, 127, 188
Commotion, 187
Con Game, 190
Concertina, 180, 182-183, 188, 191
Contessina, 72, 189
Continentalvictory, **48**
Coquelicot, 185
Corcyra, 134
Cornish Prince, 106, 124, 193
Cosmah, 146
Cosmic Bomb, 146
Cosquilla, 14, 72, 78, 80, 82, 86, 98, 100, 102, 106, 124, 189, 192-193, 195
Cosquita, 76
Coturnix, 191

Count Fleet, 72, 106, 124, 184, 189-190, 193
Count Schomberg, 189
Counterpoint, 184
Courtly Dee, 178
Cow Girl II, 150
Craig An Eran, 146
Craig Miller, 138
Creese, 184
Crepe Myrtle, 76, 78, 80, 82
Crimson Saint, 195
Crimson Satan, 195
Crispin, 50
Curiosity, 136
Cushion, 183
Cyllene, 98, 136, 154, 181, 192, 196
Daisydale D, 50
Dalmary, 187
Dame Masham, 110, 140, 154, 181
Darioletta, 194
Dark Ronald, 192, 196
Darkie, 196
Darnley, 48
Deadlock, 188
Dean Hanover, 46, 48, 52
Desert Secret, **82**
Desmond, 120, 127, 186
Devotion, 140, 142, 197
Diadumenos, 102
Dianthus, 124
Dick Andrews, 66
Dillcisco, 46
Dillciso, 52
Dimaggio, 193
Dinner Time, 58, 106
Diomed, 66
Direct Hal, 50
Discovery, 14, 58, 76, 82, 86, 106, 124, 134, 136, 150, 178-179, 184, 186-187, 190, 195
Disguise, 136, 183, 192
Display, 14, 86, 134, 136, 179, 186, 195
Djebel, 72, 86, 178
Djeddah, 72, 82, 178
Djezima, 72, 178
Dogaresa, 187
Doll Tearsheet, 110, 140
Domino, 110, 116, 127, 138, 154, 181, 188
Don John, 138
Donatella, 106
Doncaster, 110, 116, 140, 191, 197
Doremi, 154, 181-182, 188, 191
Doris, 116, 181
Double Life, 58
Double Time, 76
Doxa, 154, 181
Dr. Fager, **183**

Draymont, 183
Driver, 66
Dugout, 14, 134
Durbar II, 188
Dustwhirl, 127
Earl's Princess Martha, 46, 52
Easy Goer, **184**
Eclair, 196
Eclipse, 138
Economist, 194
Edmund, 194
Eglantine, 14, 72, 98, 100, 102, 189, 192
Eight Thirty, 106, 124, 193, 195
El Greco, 100
Elastic, 138
Eleanor, 66
Ella Brown, 50
Ellen Horne, 140
Emilia, 138, 140
Emily's Pride, 48, 52
Emily Scott, 48, 52
Emma C., 116, 127, 188
Enquirer, 138
Equipoise, 76, 80, 180
Escutcheon, 78
Espino, 76
Estoril, 185
Eternal, 183
Ethnarch, 72, 196
Eulogy, 80
Evelina, 66
Evelyn The Great, 46
Evensong, 46, 48, 52
Exalted, 146
Excamillo, 185
Excellenza, 192
Exciting Speed, 48
Expresson, 48
Fair Charmer, 76, 78, 80, 82
Fair Colleen, 195
Fair Play, 14, 100, 102, 110, 134, 136, 140, 154, 178, 180-181, 196
Fair Trial, 187
Fairvale, 195
Fairy Bridge, 82
Fairy Gold, 102, 110, 134, 136, 140, 154, 180-181
Fairy Ray, 188
Fancy Racket, 78
Fanny Dawon, 194
Fariman, 116, 154
Faugh-A-Ballagh, 138
Feola, 76, 80
Fidgette, 185
Firdaussi, 185
Firetop, 106
First Rose, 195
Flagette, 150, 185
Flambette, 188
Flambino, 188

Flaming Page, 106, 124, 193
Flaming Swords, 146
Flaming Top, 106, 124, 193
Flares, 187, 195
Flaring Top, 106, 124, 193
Fleur, 185
Flitabout, 190
Flitters, 120, 127
Floranthe, 194
Florican, 46, 52
Florimel, 46
Florine, 140
Flory Messenger, 46
Flower Bed, 100
Flower Bowl, 100
Flying Diadem, 187
Flying Duchess, 142, 191, 194, 197
Flying Dutchman, 142, 194
Flying Fox, 154, 181-182, 188, 191
Flying Witch, 146, 186
Follow Me, 46
Follow Up, 46
Forli, 82, 187
Fortino II, 58
Fota, 116, 181
Foxglove, 187
Fractious, 66
Frailty, 182
Fraxinella, 66
Free For All, 150, 183
Friar's Balsam, 182
Friar's Carse, 124
Friar Marcus, 80
Fricassee, 183
Frivolity, 191
Frizeur, 80
Gaga, 78, 86, 180, 184, 190
Gainsborough, 58, 72, 100, 120, 146, 182, 185-187, 196
Galeottia, 98
Galicia, 98, 120, 182, 196
Galla Colors, 76, 146
Gallant Fox, 188
Galliard, 110, 140, 191
Gallice, 134
Gallinule, 98, 102, 116, 120, 127, 189, 192
Galopin, 98, 116, 120, 140, 142, 182, 191, 194, 197
Gay Crusader, 14, 72, 98, 100, 102, 189, 192
Gay Forbes, 50
Gay Gamp, 100
Gay Girl Chimes, 50
Gay Laura, 98, 102, 189, 192

Gay Missile, 86
Geisha, 82, 106, 124, 136, 178-179, 184, 186-187, 190, 195
Giantess, 66
Glacier, 182
Gladiator, 138
Glamour, 76, 78, 80, 82
Glare, 98
Glasalt, 182
Glencoe, 66, 194
Gnat, 183
Gohanna, 66
Gohanna Mare, 66
Gold Bridge, 187
Gold Digger, 190
Gold Girl, 50
Golden Boss, 187
Goldfinch, 188
Gondolette, 182, 196
Good Goods, 76, 80
Good Note, 48, 52
Goody Two Shoes, 120, 127
Graustark, 100
Great Above, 150
Grey Dawn II, 150, **185**
Grey Leg, 98, 102, 189, 192
Grey Sovereign, 58
Guiccioli, 194
Guiding Star, 187
Guy Axworthy, 46, 50
Guy Dillon, 50
Guy McKinney, 46
Hail To Reason, 76, 78, 82, 146
Hal Dale, 50
Halo, 146
Hampton, 110, 116, 120, 140, 188, 191
Hanover's Bertha, 46
Hanover Maid, 46
Harkaway, 142, 194
Harmonicon, 14, 192
Harpalice, 66
Harpsichord, 192
Harry Of Hereford, 102, 110, 154, 180, 181
Harvest Gale, 46
Hassock, 183
Haste, 72, 189
Hastings, 102, 110, 134, 136, 140, 154, 180-181
Hasty Girl, 116
Hasty Road, 190
Hautesse II, 136
Havresac II, 14, 72, 134, 186-187
Heather Bell, 116
Hedge Rose, 138
Heelfly, 58
Hegira, 138
Heldifann, 72

Helene De Troie, 154, 180-181, 183
Helicon, 154, 180-181
Hemlock, 134, 136
Herbager, 150, 185
Hermit, 116, 140, 142, 197
Herod Mare, 66
Herodiade, 146, 189
Herodias, 146, 189
Hickory Pride, 48, 52
Hickory Smoke, 48
Highflyer, 66
Highflyer Mare, 66
Hildene, 78
Hill Prince, 78
Himyar, 110, 127, 138
Hi-Nelli, 76
Hippodrome, 181
Hira, 138
His Majesty, 134, 136
Holy Bull, 150
Honor Bright, 48
Honora, 189
Hoot Mon, 46, 48, 52
Hornsea, 194
Hors Concours, 134, 186
Hostess, 46
Hour Glass II, 136
Humanity, 179
Hurakan, 78, 102
Hurry On, 58, 182
Hydroplane II, 182
Hyperion, 72, 82, 100, 106, 179, 182, 186-187, 195-196
I Will, 150
Iago, 138
Illuminata, 188
Immortelle, 116
Imperatrice, 14, 82, 86, 192, 195
Imprint, 124
In Prime Time, 193
In The Purple, 124
Indian Hemp, 58, 193
Indolence, 14, 72, 80, 86, 98, 100, 102, 106, 189, 192
Infra Red, 72, 106
Inheritor, 194
Intent, 150
Intentionally, 150
Intercontinental, 48
Ion, 142, 194
Iron Maiden, 196
Iron Reward, 196
Irony, 191
Isabel, 120
Isette, 14, 192
Isinglass, 98, 110, 120, 127, 182, 188, 192
Isoletta, 120
Isonomy, 98, 116, 188
Ivy Leaf, 110, 127, 138

Jabot, 184
Jack High, 124
Jamestown, 58
Jean Claire, 50
Jen Hanover, 52
Jerboa, 194
Jet Action, 76, 78, 80, 82
Jet Pilot, 76, 78, 80, 82
Joe Andrews, 66
John O'Gaunt, 110, 120, 127, 154, 181
John P. Grier, 76, 136, 179, 186
Johnstown, 184, 190
Josephine Brewer, 46
Josephine Knight, 46
Judy O'Grady, 185
Judy-Rae, 178
June Rose, 14, 192
Juniper, 194
Just-A-Minute, 193
Kampala, 100
Karen's Choice, 48, 52
Karenza, 196
Kentucky, 138
Key Bridge, 100, **102**
Key To The Mint, 100
Keystone Starlet, 46
Khaled, 196
King Fergus, 66
King Tom, 140, 142, 191, 194, 197
Knight's Daughter, 76, 78, 80, 82
Knockaney Bridge, 72
Knowsley, 191
Kong, 58
L'Abesse De Jouarre, 120, 127
La Chica, 136, 179, 186
La Dorette, 197
La Farina, 185
La Flambee, 188
La Fleche, 110, 120, 127, 196
La Grisette, 136
La Mome, 190
La Troienne, 72, 78, 80, 86, 154, 180-181, 183-184, 190
Lacerta, 194
Ladas, 196
Lady Angela, 82, 106, 124, 186-187, 193, 195
Lady Brilliant, 196
Lady Cicero, 180
Lady Comfey, 179
Lady Emily, 191
Lady Erectress, 50
Lady Erne, 179
Lady Evelyn, 142, 197
Lady Glory, 178-179, 184, 190
Lady Hamburg II, 183

Lady Josephine, 14, 72, 120, 134, 185
Lady Langden, 140
Lady Langdon, 191
Lady Lawless, 86
Lady Lightfoot, 98, 102, 136, 189, 192
Lady Martha, 98
Lady Masham, 140
Lady Of Pedigree, 154, 180-181
Lady Of The Snows, 58
Lady Villikins, 98, 182
Lalun, 72, 82, 178
Lark Hanover, 52
Larksnest, 58
Lassie Dear, 86
Laughing Dream, 180
Laura, 191
Laura Gal, 190
Lauretta, 116
Laurita Hanover, 48, 52
Lavendula, 146
Laveno, 116, 154
Lawful Tip, 52
Le Samaritain, 120
Leamington, 138
Leda, 194
Lee Tide, 46
Leta Long, 50
Lexington, 138, 140
Lida, 138
Life Hill, 58
Light Brigade, 14, 134, 136
Lily Agnes, 127, 197
Little Fairy, 142, 194
Liz F., 150
Lizzie G., 138
Loika, 72
Lord Clifden, 140, 142, 191, 197
Lord Lyon, 191
Lou Sidney, 48
Loved One, 116
Lowland Chief, 182
Lucy Abbey, 48
Lygie, 188
Macaroni, 116, 140, 191, 197
MacGregor, 110, 140
Mackeath, 116
Mafosta, 193
Mah Mahal, 120, 146, 150, 185-187
Mahmoud, 82, 100, 106, **120**, 146, 150, 185-187, 195
Mahubah, 100, 102, 110, 140, 154, 178, 180-181, 196
Maid Marian, 136, 192, 196
Maid Of Erin, 188

Maid Of Palmyra, 142, 197
Maid Of The Mint, 110, 182, 188, 191
Maintenant, 189
Malachite, 189
Malatesta, 185
Malcolm Forbes, 50
Malva, 14, 72, 80, 120, 127, 134, 146, 185-186
Man O' War, 78, 80, 86, 100, 102, 110, 124, **140**, 146, 154, 178-181, 183-185, 190, 196
Mandy Hamilton, 180
Manganese, 142
Manna, 58, 110, 140
Mannie Gray, 110, 138
Mannie Grey, 127
Marching Home, 76, 78
Marco, 98, 182
Marcovil, 98, 102, 182, 189, 192
Margaret, 194
Margaret Hal, 50
Margaret Polk, 50
Marguerite, 188
Maria, 66
Marigold, 140
Market Wise, 184
Marking Time, 184
Marliacea, 120, 127
Marmion, 66
Marpessa, 66, 194
Marsyas, 142, 197
Martagon, 120, 127
Mary Seaton, 98
Masque, 188
Mata Hari, 58, 195
Matchmaker, 196
Maud, 138
Mavis, 140
Mavourneen, 182, 188
May B, 50
May Pole, 98
May Queen, 191
Mazurka, 116
Meadow Cheer, 50
Meddler, 188
Medeah, 188
Medora, 194
Melton, 188
Mendocita, 50
Menow, 78, 86, 106, 124, 180, 184, 190, 193, 195
Mercury, 66
Mercury Mare, 66
Mercy, 150
Merope, 142, 194
Merry Dance, 182
Merry Gal, 98, 102, 120, 127, 189, 192
Merry Hampton, 110, 140, 154, 181

Merry Token, 102, 110, 140, 154, 180-181
Mersey, 191
Messe, 150
Mieuxce, 150, 187
Mighty Margaret, 52
Milan Mill, 72, 106, 124, 193
Millicent, 106, 124, 193
Mill Reef, 72
Mimi Hanover, 46, 48
Mimzy, 46
Mincemeat, 140
Mindful, 14, 72, 98, 100, 102, 189, 192
Mineral, 142, 197
Minnesota Mac, 150
Minoru, 98, 102, 182, 189, 192, 196
Mint Sauce, 191
Minting, 191
Misfortune, 66
Miss Agnes, 191
Miss Carmie, 58
Miss De Forest, 46
Miss Disco, 14, 58, 76, 78, 82, 86, 106, 124, 134, 193, 195
Miss Dogwood, 190
Miss Ellah, 50
Miss Fiora, 136
Miss Gay Girl, 50
Miss Larksfly, 58
Miss Malaprop, 189
Miss Matty, 14, 72, 98, 100, 102, 189, 192
Miss Puzzle, 183
Miss Roland, 138
Miss Rushin, 58, 124, 178-179, 184
Miss Saginaw, 50
Miss Sellon, 142
Miss Tooley, 194
Missey, 46
Missile Toe, 48, 52
Missy Baba, 86
Misty Hanover, 48, 52
Miyako, 124, 136, 178-179, 184, 186-187, 190
Mizpah, 110, 140, 154, 181
Mon Etoile, 197
Monarque, 197
Monie Rosa, 138
Monte Rosa, 127
Monte Rose, 110
Moorhen, 98, 116
Moscow Ballet, **106**, 124, 193
Mother Goose, 146, 186-187
Mother Siegel, 98
Mother-In-Law, 196
Mr. McElwyn, 46, 50, 52
Mr. Music, 58

Mr. Prospector, 190
Mrs. Ridgway, 142, 194
Mulatto, 194
Mulberry, 116
Muley, 66, 194
Mumtaz Begum, 14, 58, 72, 76, 80, 82, 86, 106, 134, 146, 178-179, 184, 187, 190, 195
Mumtaz Mahal, 14, 72, 80, 86, 120, 134, 146, 178-179, 185-186
Musket, 182, 191
Mustang, 150
My Babu, 86
My Birthday, 52
My Charmer, 76, 78, **80**, 82
My Recipe, 150
My Tip, 48, 52
Myram, 192
Myrobella, 58
Myrtle Charm, 76, 78, 80, 82
Myrtlewood, 76, 80, 190
Nabocklish, 194
Nan Darrell, 194
Nancy Hanks, 50
Nantallah, 82, 187
Napolean Direct, 50
Napoli, 116
Nashua, 190
Nasrullah, 14, 58, 72, 76, 78, 80, 82, 86, 106, 124, 134, 178-179, 184, 187, 190, 193, 195
Nassocian, 134
Nassovian, 136
Natalma, 82, 106, 124, 186-187, 193, 195
Native Dancer, 82, 106, 124, **136**, 178-179, 184, 186-187, 190, 193, 195
Navarra, 58
Nearco, 14, 58, 72, 76, 80, 82, 86, 106, 124, 134, 146, 178-179, 184, 186-187, 190, 193, 195
Nearctic, 82, 106, 124, 186-187, 193, 195
Necklace, 140
Necromancer, 116
Neddie, 80
Needles, 124
Nell, 194
Nelly Zarro, 50
Neptunus, 138
Nervesa, 58
Nervolo Belle, 50
Nevele Pride, 48
Never Bend, 72, 178
New Providence, 195
Newminster, 142, 197
Nijinsky II, 106, 124, 193

Noble Chieftain, 98
Noble Martha, 98, 102, 189, 192
Noble Victory, 48, 52
Nogara, 14, 72, 80, 82, 86, 106, 134, 146, 178-179, 186-187, 195
Noisette, 66
Nonpareil, 183
Noodle Soup, 124
Nopro Blama, 193
North Star II, 116
North Star III, 102, 154, 180-181, 189
Northern Dancer, 82, 106, 124, **186-187**, 193, 195
Not Afraid, 189
Nothirdchance, 76, 78, 82, 146
Nureyev, 187
Occult, 106
Omaha, 106, **188**
On Hand, 184
On The Move, 193
On-And-On, 178-179, 184
Oola Hills, 193
Ophirdale, 127
Oreen, 183
Orlando, 197
Orme, 98, 191, 197
Ormonda, 127
Ormonde, 127, 191, 197
Orsenigo, 58
Orville, 66
Our Lassie, 196
Our Page, 106, 124, 193, 195
Outdone, 14, 58, 76, 82, 86, 106, 134, 195
Over There, 146, 189
Owen Tudor, 150
Oxford, 138
Padilla, 116, 154
Padua, 116, 154
Padula, 102, 116, 154, 180, 189
Page Book, 124
Palotta, 120
Panasette, 183
Panasine, 183
Panay, 150, 183
Pankhurst, 183
Papalona, 195
Papila, 195
Pappa Fourway, 193
Pappageno II, 193
Papyrus, 14, 72, 80, 86, 98, 100, 102, 106, 189, 192
Paradox, 182
Pasquil, 136, 192
Pasquita, 14, 136, 192
Paul Jones, 116
Pauline, 110, 140

Paulowitz, 194
Pavot, 185
Peace, 146, 186
Peace Chance, 146, 186, 187
Peace Corps, 52
Penelope, 66
Penicuik II, 179
Pennant, 80, 180
Pensive, 58, 124, 178-179, 184
Pepper And Salt, 98
Perdita II, 98
Perfume II, 86
Perlette, 150
Permission, 110
Persimmon, 98, 102, 136, 189, 192
Pert Flirt, 48
Perth, 98, 102, 189, 192
Peter Pan, 116, 154, 183
Peter Scott, 50
Peter Song, 46
Peter The Great, 46, 50
Peter Volo, 46, 50
Petrarch, 191
Petrex, 46
Phalaris, 14, 72, 134, 136, 146, 180, 185-187
Pharamond II, 78, 86, 106, 146, 180, 184, 190
Pharis, 106
Pharos, 14, 72, 80, 82, 86, 100, 106, 134, 146, 178-179, 185-187, 195
Phideas, 150
Philomath, 98
Phonograph, 52
Photinia, 116
Picton, 134, 136
Pietra, 192
Pilate, 106
Pilgrimage, 110, 120, 127
Pillow Talk, 52
Pink Domino, 102, 110, 127, 136, 138, 154, 180-181
Pitti, 189
Pladda, 185
Plaisanterie, 98, 197
Planutess, 196
Plassy, 185
Plucky Liege, 146, 180, 182-183, 188, 191, 196
Plum Cake, 178-179, 184
Pocahontas, 66, 142, 194, 197
Poetess, 197
Poker, 76, 78, 80, 82
Polamia, 150, 185
Polly Agnes, 197
Polly Parrot, 50
Polymelian, 14, 86, 136, 179, 186, 192

Polymelus, 14, 134, 136, 146, 180, 186, 192, 196
Polynesian, 76, 78, 82, 106, 124, 136, 178-179, 184, 186-187, 190, 193, 195
Pompey, 14, 86, 134, 136
Ponder, 58, 124, 178-179, 184
Pot Eight O's, 66
Precipitation, 58
Preciptic, 195
Pretty Does, 184
Primrose Dame, 98
Prince John, 189
Prince Palatine, 14, 72, 98, 100, 102, 136, 189, 192
Prince Rose, 14, 72, 76, 78, 80, 82, 86, 98, 100, 102, 106, 124, 189, 192-193, 195
Princequillo, 14, 72, 76, 78, 80, 82, 86, **98**, 100, 102, 124, 189, 192, 193, 195
Princess Catherine, 191
Protector, 46
Prunella, 66
Queen Mary, 138
Queenly McKinney, 46
Questionnaire, 150, 183
Quetta, 98
Quick Thought, 14, 72, 80, 86, 98, 100, 102, 106, 189, 192
Quickly, 72, 106, 140, 189-190
Rabelais, 134, 186, 188
Rackety Coo, 192
Radium, 188
Raise A Native, 178-179, 184, 190
Raise You, 178-179, 184, 190
Rampart, 124
Ranavalo III, 58
Rare Bloom, 195
Rataplan, 142
Real Delight, 178-179, 184
Reason To Earn, 76, 78
Red Ray, 72, 106, 124, 193
Reform, 110, 127, 138
Regal Roman, 180
Reigh Count, 72, 106, 189-190
Relaxing, 184
Relic, 58
Requiebro, 195
Ribbon, 138
Ribot, 100
Right-Away, 98
Riot, 187

Risky, 100, 102
Risque, 100, 102
Risque Blue, 100, 102
Robert Le Diable, 120, 127, 188
Rock Sand, 98, 102, 110, 136, 140, **142**, 154, 180-181, 189, 192, 197
Rodney, 46, 48, 52
Roi Herode, 120, 134, 136, 180, 192, 196
Roman, 150, 190
Romanella, 100
Rondeau, 154, 179-183, 188, 191-192
Roquebrune, 98, 110, 140, 142, 154, 181, 197
Rosalinda, 48
Rosaline, 120, 182, 196
Rosalys, 120
Rose Bay, 120, 127, 188
Rose De Mai, 98, 102, 189, 192
Rose Eternal, 183
Rose Leaves, 106, 179, 182
Rose Of Lancaster, 188
Rose Of Roses, 183
Rose Prince, 14, 72, 80, 86, 98, 100, 102, 106, 189, 192
Rose Scott, 50
Rosedrop, 120, 182, 185-186, 196
Rosemary Hanover, 52
Rosette, 50
Roseville, 110, 116, 127, 138, 154, 181
Rothesay Bay, 185
Rouge Et Noir, 146
Rouge Rose, 110, 116, 140, 191, 197
Rough'n Tumble, 150, 183
Rough Shod II, 82, 187
Round Table, 76, 78, 80, 82
Roused, 150, 183
Roxelane, 120
Roya McKinney, 50
Royal Charger, 76, 86, 146
Ruby Nethersole, 183
Rude Awakening, 150, 183
Rustorm Mahal, 150
Sabella, 193
Sabzy, 58, 193
Sadler's Wells, 82
Sailing Home, 76, 78
Sainfoin, 98, 110, 140, 142, 154, 181-182, 197
Saltram, 66
Samphire, 188
San Francisco, 50

Sanda, 110, 140, 142, 197
Sandal, 120, 127, 140, 142, 197
Sandbeck, 194
Sandy Flash, 46
Sans Souci II, 185
Sarita, 186-187
Satirical, 188
Saumur, 191
Scandal, 138
Scapa Flow, 14, 72, 134, 186-187
Sceptical, 195
Scotch Love, 46, 52
Scotland, 46, 52
Sea Gull, 138
Seattle Slew, 76, 78
Seclusion, 142, 197
Secretariat, 14, 82, 86, 195
Seeking The Gold, 190
Segula, 190
Sekhmet, 190
Selene, 72, 100, 136, 146, 180, 182, 186-187, 196
Selim, 66
Selka Guy, 46
Selka Scot, 46
Sequence, 190
Seraph, 188
Serengati, 150
Serenissima, 136, 146, 180, 182, 185-186, 196
Seven Thirty, 58
Sharon Brown, 150
Shimmer, 187
Shining Sun, 195
Shut Out, 150
Sibola, 134, 186
Sickle, 136, 179, 186
Sierra, 116, 120
Sigrid Volo, 50
Simon's Shoes, 187
Simonath, 98, 102, 189, 192
Sir Cosmo, 76, 80
Sir Gallahad III, 78, 80, 146, 178, 188, 190-**191**, 196
Sir Gaylord, 86
Sir Hercules, 194
Sir Peter, 66
Sissy's Time, 124
Sister Sarah, 82, 106, 186-187, 195
Sister To Adonis, 138
Sister To Eve, 140
Sister To Ouida, 138
Sister To Pan, 138
Skylark, 191
Slew O' Gold, 78
Snowberry, 58
Solario, 58, 146, 185
Somethingroyal, 14, 82, 86, **192**, 195

Somolli, 48, 52
Son-In-Law, 100, 178, 185, 196
Source Sucree, 76, 86, 146
South Ocean, 195
Soviet Problem, 193
Spearmint, 110, 134, 154, 180-183, 186, 188-189, 191
Special, 82, 187
Speedster, 46, 48, 52
Speedy Crown, 48, 52
Speedy Scot, 46, 48, 52
Speedy Somolli, 48, 52
Spencer, 46
Spencer Scott, 46, 52
Spendthrift, 110, 140, 154, 181
Spicebox, 185
Springfield, 110, 140, 142, 197
Spud Hanover, 46
Spur, 183
Spy Song, 195
St. Albans, 140, 142, 197
St. Angela, 140, 142, 182, 191, 194, 197
St. Angelo, 116, 181
St. Denis, 154, 181
St. Frusquin, 120, 182, 188, 196
St. Germany, 146
St. Marguerite, 110, 140, 142, 197
St. Marina, 188
St. Simon, 98, 110, 120, 127, 140, 142, 182, 188, 191, **194**, 196-197
Star, 182
Star's Pride, 46, 48, 52
Stardrift, 46, 48, 52
Stefan The Great, 189
Stephanie, 72, 189
Stepwisely, 195
Sterling, 138
Stimulus, 78, 100, 102
Sting, 183
Stockwell, 140, 142, 197
Stolen Kisses, 138
Storm Bird, 195
Storm Cat, 195
Striking, 76, 78, 80, 82, 193
Sugar Frosting, 48, 52
Sultan, 66, 194
Summer Girl, 110, 154, 181, 189
Sun Again, 195
Sun Briar, 14, 134, 136, 180
Sun Princess, 146
Sun Worship, 58

Sundridge, 110, 116, 120, 134, 136, 181, 189, 192, 196
Sunreigh, 72, 189
Sunshine, 116
Sunstar, 116, 154, 181
Super Bowl, 52
Superman, 127
Supremus, 180
Supromene, 124
Swaps, 196
Sweep, 100, 102, 110, 127, 134, 136, **138**, 154, 178, 180-181, 196
Sweep On, 14, 134
Sweep Out, 14, 86, 134
Sweet Briar II, 134, 189
Sweet Lavender, 146
Sweet Music, 14, 86, 192
Sweet Tooth, 178-179, 184
Sweetheart, 178-179, 184-185, 190
Swinging, 80, 180
Swynford, 120, 127, 134, 185-186
T.V. Lark, 58
Ta Wee, 150
Tadmor, 142
Taia, 188
Tar Heel, 50
Tarport Cheer, 50
Tartlet, 140
Tea Caddy, 183
Teak, 183
Teddy, 14, 146, 154, 178-180-185, 188, 190-192, 196
Teleran, 106, 124, 193
Tellaris, 106, 124, 193
Tenerani, 100
Tenserino, 193
Teresina, 100
Terlingua, 195
Termagent, 66
Thankful, 48
Thankful Blossom, 182
The Abbe, 50
The Apple, 182
The Axe II, 150
The Baron, 142
The Boss, 80
The Intruder, 48, 52
The Last Red, 124
The Porter, 179
The Ranger, 197
The Slave, 142
The Slayer's Daughter, 140
The Tetrarch, 14, 72, 120, 134, 185, 189, 196
Thong, 82, 187
Thormanby, 140
Tibthorpe or Cremorne, 116

Tilly Kate, 150, 183
Tilly Rose, 150, 183
Time To Dine, 58
Tisma Hanover, 48
Titan Hanover, 48
To Market, 184
Toboggan, 182
Tofanella, 100
Tom Fool, 78, 86, 180, 184, 190, 193
Tom Kendle, 50
Tomahawk, 110, 140
Topiary, 98, 102, 189, 192, 197
Tosca, 48
Touchstone, 142
Tourbillon, 72
Tout Suite, 182
Toxophilite, 191
Trace Call, 124
Tracery, 14, 72, 98, 100, 102, 186, 189, 192, **197**
Traffic, 190
Traffic Court, 190
Tramp, 66
Trampoline, 66, 194
Trenton, 120, 182
Trevisa, 82, 187
Tristan, 110, 120, 127
Trocadero, 197
Trumpator, 66
Try Try Again, 100
Tulle, 178
Turn-To, 76, 78, 82, 86, 146
Twice Over, 58
Twilight Hanover, 48
Two Bob, 58, 178-179, 184
Two Lea, 178-179, 184
Twosy, 58
Ultimus, 78, 102, 179-180
Umidwar, 86
Unbreakable, 76, 124, 136, 178-179, 184, 186-187, 190
Uncas or Thurio, 116
Uncle, 196
Uncle's Lassie, 178, 196
Under Fire, 134
Underhand, 140
Upset, 183
Urania, 188
Uvira II, 86
Vahren, 120, 134, 196
Vaila, 102, 116, 154, 180, 189
Vain Duchess, 154, 181
Valdina Moza, 193
Valley Victoria, 48
Valley Victory, 48
Vampire, 191
Vandale, 150, 185
Vanille, 185
Vaya, 185

Vedette, 142, 191, 194, 197
Velocipede's Dam, 194
Veneta, 187
Venturesome II, 102
Verona, 116
Victorious Lou, 48
Victory Song, 46, 48, 52
Villamor, 124
Virginia Water, 72, 124, 193
Viridis, 140, 142, 197
Volomite, 46, 48, 50, 52
Voltaire, 194
Voltigeur, 142, 194
Voter, 182
Wait A Bit, 76, 78

Walter Direct, 50
War Admiral, 76, 78, 80, 86, 100, 102, **110**, 154, 178, 180-181, 183-184, 190, 196
War Dance, 98, 138
War Relic, 58, 124, 150
Warble, 191
Warrior Lass, 76
Warwell Worthy, 46, 52
Waterhen, 185
Waxy, 66
Web, 66
Weekend Surprise, 86
Wellingtonia, 191, 197
Wenlock, 140, 142, 197
West Australian, 138, 140

Whirlaway, 127
Whisk Broom II, 136, 179, 183
Whisker, 194
Whiskey, 66
Whisper, 138
White Eagle, 14, 72, 98, 100, 102, 120, 127, 189, 192
Widow Maggie, 50
Wild Arum, 120, 127, 134, 185
Wildair, 80, 183
William The Third, 196
Williamson's Ditto, 66
Wilmington, 50
Winds Chant, 76, 80

Winning Colors, 58
Wonder, 136
Woodbine, 138
Woodpecker, 66
Worth A Plenty, 52
Worth Beein', 52
Worth Seein, 52
Worthy Boy, 46, 48, 52
Wrack, 188
Xanthina, 150
Yodler, 134
Young Giantess, 66
Young Noisette, 66
Your Host, 124
Zodiac, 194

Entries in bold face indicate featured pedigrees